Ethnicity and Fertility in Southeast Asia Series
General Editors: Aline K. Wong and Ng Shui Meng

ETHNICITY AND FERTILITY IN THAILAND

by

Suchart Prasithrathsint

Research Notes and Discussions Paper No. 51
INSTITUTE OF SOUTHEAST ASIAN STUDIES
1985

Published by
Institute of Southeast Asian Studies
Heng Mui Keng Terrace
Pasir Panjang
Singapore 0511

ISSN 0129-8828
ISBN 9971-988-13-5

CONTENTS

Page

LIST OF TABLES

Page

Page

Page

Page

LIST OF FIGURES

MAP

ACKNOWLEDGEMENTS

The study of ethnicity and fertility in Thailand is part of the five ASEAN countries' project on ethnicity and fertility. The Thai study covers 4 major ethnic groups living in all major regions of the country. The total sample consists of 858 Thai, 837 Chinese, 838 Thai Muslim and 587 Southern Thai Muslim couples. The study is the first of its kind dealing empirically with a wide range of social, economic, and demographic characteristics of the major ethnic groups and their ethnic relations. The findings of the research project are not only very informative but also full of policy implications. The Thai study has contributed a great deal to the understanding of the ways of life of the four ethnic groups and their fertility and family planning behaviour.

The research project would have been impossible without a substantial amount of financial support from the Rockefeller Foundation. We duly wish to express our gratitude to the Rockefeller Foundation, and in particular to Dr Mary Kritz. We also wish to thank the National Institute of Development Administration for providing supplementary financial support for the project. I personally wish to thank my co-investigators in various regions of the country: Assistant Professor Luechai Chulasai, Chiangmai University; Assistant Professor Thawatchai Arthorn-thurasook, Mahidol University; Archan Laddawan Rodmanee, Mahidol University; Assistant Professor Saranya Bunnag, Prince of Songkla University; and Associate Professor Suwanlee Piampiti, the National Institute of Development Administration, for their participation in field data collection and international workshops on the project.

My thanks are also due to Miss Laurie Rosenthal of the Nation Review, who helped edit the research report.

Suchart Prasithrathsint

PREFACE

The Ethnicity and Fertility in Southeast Asia Project that commenced in 1980, was an outgrowth of an earlier project, Culture and Fertility in Southeast Asia, which was completed in 1979. Building upon the results of the earlier study, which established that ethnicity was a significant factor underlying the fertility differentials among the various ethnic groups in Southeast Asia, the present project aimed to explore in greater detail the extent to which ethnicity and ethnic factors like ethnic attitudes, ethnic identification and cultural practices influenced reproductive behaviour. Instead of utilizing secondary sources, the project relied on primary data collected through the survey technique. In all, twenty ethnic groups from the five ASEAN countries were surveyed in this study which spanned a total of three years.

A study involving five different countries and so many ethnic groups of diverse cultural and religious backgrounds would invariably pose problems of comparability. To maximize comparability across countries, the study relied on the use of a common core questionnaire as well as a common analytical framework and data analysis procedures. While comparability was important, the incorporation of country-specific factors salient and relevant to the explanation of fertility behaviour was also encouraged. The final research design therefore attempted to be as comprehensive as possible in the exploration of the ethnic dimension in fertility differentials among the various ethnic groups studied.

Three workshops were held during the period of the project to enable the researchers to come together to discuss and resolve problems related to the project. The first workshop was held in May 1980. At this workshop the conceptual framework and the core questionnaire were finalized. In the second workshop held in June 1981, the methods of data analysis were decided. At the final workshop in September 1982, the country teams presented their preliminary findings. The final reports were completed by December 1983.

A study of this scale obviously also involved many researchers. The researchers were all Southeast Asian social scientists drawn from various disciplines and backgrounds. Some were attached to universities of the region while others were from research institutes or government agencies.

Dr Rodolfo A. Bulatao from the East-West Population Institute provided the initial intellectual impetus to the project by formulating the conceptual framework and research design for the study as well as the drafting of the preliminary questionnaire. In addition Dr Bulatao together with Dr Aline K. Wong from the National University of Singapore (NUS) and Dr Ng Shui Meng from ISEAS served as co-ordinators of the project. The country teams consisted of:

Indonesia: Dr Mely Tan (National Institute of Economic and Social Research of the Indonesian Institute of Sciences, LEKNAS-LIPI)

Dr Budi Soeradji (Central Bureau of Statistics)

Mr Amri Marzali (Faculty of Letters, University of Indonesia)

Malaysia: Datin Dr Noor Laily Abu Bakar (Malaysia National Family Planning Board, NFPB)

Dr Tan Boon Ann (NFPB)

Mr Tey Nai Peng (NFPB)

Mr Hew Wai Sin (NFPB)

Ms Aminah Abdul Rahman (NFPB)

Ms Ramlah Haji Muda (NFPB)

Ms Nazileh Ramli (NFPB)

Mr Khalipah Mohd Tora (NFPB)

Mr Ng Tuck Seng (NFPB)

Philippines: Ms Pilar Ramos-Jimenez (Philippine Social Science Council, PSSC)

	Ms Ma. Cecilia Gastardo-Conaco (University of the Philippines)
	Ms Lorna Makil (PSSC)
	Ms Ruth N. Barniego (PSSC)
Singapore:	Dr Eddie C.Y. Kuo (National University of Singapore, NUS)
	Dr Chiew Seen-Kong (NUS)
Thailand:	Dr Suchart Prasithrathsint (National Institute of Development Administration, NIDA)
	Dr Suwanlee Piampiti (NIDA)
	Mr Thawatchai Arthorn-thurasook (Mahidol University)
	Dr Laddawan Rodmanee (Mahidol University)
	Dr Luechai Chulasai (Chiangmai University)
	Ms Suranya Bunnag (Prince of Songkla University)
	Ms Amporn Chareonchai (Khon Kaen University)

Funding for the project was provided by the International Development Research Centre (IDRC), Rockefeller Foundation and the Human Reproduction Programme, Task Force on Psychosocial Research in Family Planning of the World Health Organization (WHO).

The results of the study are being published in six monographs in this series:

Ethnicity and Fertility in Southeast Asia: A Comparative Analysis

Ethnicity and Fertility in Indonesia

Ethnicity and Fertility in Malaysia

Ethnicity and Fertility in the Philippines

Ethnicity and Fertility in Singapore

Ethnicity and Fertility in Thailand

ALINE WONG and NG SHUI MENG
Project Co-ordinators
and
General Editors of the Series

I

INTRODUCTION

Fertility is indeed an extremely complex demographic phenomenon. The decision to have children is made by millions of couples with different ways of life, orientations, life goals and social situations. In addition, all these things are, in turn, related to or affected by a multitude of changing social, political, economic, psychological, cultural and physiological factors. An attempt to understand the fertility of a human population is further complicated by the existence of various ethnic groups with different cultural and social traits and by the nature of the inter-ethnic group relationships. A thorough understanding of fertility in an ethnically diverse society cannot be achieved without analysing the relationships between ethnicity and fertility.

The present study represents one of the earliest studies of the relationship of ethnicity and fertility. In fact, it can claim to be the first of its kind to focus on the issue with a national survey specifically designed for the purpose. It was preceded by a much smaller pilot project, entitled "Culture and Fertility: The Case of Thailand" (Prasithrathsint, et al., 1980).

The term "ethnicity" in this research is used in a broad sense to cover identification of individuals by race, religion, language, nationality and similar primordial characteristics.

Purposes of the Study

Thailand is an ethnically diverse country, even though the majority of its population are Thai. There are two major distinct minority groups -- the Thai Muslims and the Chinese.

The main purposes of the research project are to study the nature of fertility differentials among the Thais, the Chinese and the Thai Muslims and to identify the causes of differentials or factors affecting them.

Similar research projects have also been conducted by other members of ASEAN countries. The common objectives of these research projects are: (1) to provide a systematic, comparative description of ethnic differentials in fertility and associated cultural practices in the five ASEAN countries; (2) to attempt to explain the differentials within a multivariate framework; (3) to assess the effect of fertility differentials in perceptions of ethnic relations; (4) to suggest policies for dealing with ethnic differentials in the countries studied; and (5) to provide training, as part of the research process, to junior members of the research teams. Each of these objectives may be considered further.

Systematic description: There have been no previous attempts to provide systematic, comparative descriptions of ethnic differentials in fertility across the ASEAN countries. Such a description should stimulate thought about country parallels and contrasts; how ethnicity functions in different contexts; and the types of barriers between ethnic groups that may impede fertility decline. The aim of this project is to provide a cross-sectional description, although comparisons may be made with historical data from other sources. The description should cover not only fertility measures but also related cultural practices. The description should also involve looking at differentials across social class, age and residential groups as these relate to ethnic differentials.

Explanations for differentials: The second objective is to take the differentials that have been described and attempt to explain them. Evaluating the hypotheses listed is part of this process. These hypotheses are merely illustrative, however, and the objective is to investigate as many factors as possible within the general framework. The goal is a simplified framework eliminating the factors that have little or no effect, but adding indicators of the relative importance of the factors that remain. Such a framework should then be able to account for ethnic differentials within each country.

Fertility and ethnic relations: Ethnic differentials in fertility exist in a political context and are a factor in ethnic relations. The existence of ethnic differentials raises not only scientific questions about actual causes but also political questions about how people react to differentials. An attempt is made to determine perceptions of, beliefs about, and attitudes toward ethnic differentials at the individual level. Such subjective reactions are coloured by inter-ethnic attitudes, which are therefore also studied. We seek to determine how people feel about the differentials they perceive and how these feelings relate to other inter-ethnic attitudes.

Policy implications: After the previous objectives are satisfied, an attempt is made to draw implications for population policy from the results. Ethnicity itself is not a policy variable: it is generally not subject to manipulation. However, this project attempts to go beyond ethnic labels and identify those aspects of ethnic subcultures and group social positions related to fertility. These factors may be more amenable to control, or at least deserve more sympathetic treatment. The findings resulting from the study will contribute to the understanding of fertility of different ethnic groups in the country. It is expected that with the knowledge and awareness of ethnic fertility differentials and factors affecting them, the population and development policy-makers can formulate population policies and programmes more acceptable to the ethnic groups covered by the present study. Different appeals and approaches for each ethnic group or work with the critical cultural and social factors affecting fertility of specific groups may be developed.

Training: For this project, a research team was organized to cover each country. Each team generally had one senior researcher with survey experience and one or more junior researchers with less training. Given the limited social-scientific resources in the countries under study, it would have been impractical -- besides unnecessary -- to involve a larger number of senior researchers. The project was, however, to serve the subsidiary objective of providing valuable research experience, within the context of a carefully designed cross-cultural investigation, for the junior researchers.

Studies of Ethnic Fertility Differentials in Thailand

Based on the broad definition of ethnicity specified earlier, there are a few studies done in Thailand. A study of religious fertility differentials based on the 1960 census data found that religious fertility differentials did exist (Goldstein 1970). According to the study, women who professed to subscribe to Confucian beliefs had slightly more children than Buddhists, while both these groups averaged considerably more children than did Moslem women. A recent pilot study of the ethnic fertility differentials in Bangkok found the contrary. The Moslem had the highest fertility followed by the Thai and the Chinese respectively. However, the differences became less when the analysis was controlled for differences in place of residence, education of wife and husband, household income, female labour-force participation, marriage duration and woman's current age. More recently a comparative study of factors affecting a desire for a two-child family of the Thai Buddhist and the Thai Moslems was conducted in Southern Thailand. It was found that the Thai Buddhist were more receptive to family planning and a two-child family than the Thai Moslems (Bunnag 1982).

Related to the studies of ethnic fertility differentials are studies of other fertility differentials or studies of factors affecting the fertility behaviour of the Thai families without taking into account the ethnicity of the household heads and their spouses. There are numerous studies of the kind. Many of them analysed factors that are included in the present study. They, for instance, include the studies of general fertility levels and differentials in Thailand, the influence of female labour force participation, and education (Goldstein 1972), and the fertility threshold value of education and income (Prasithrathsint 1979), son preference (Prasithrathsint 1972), religiosity (Prompaichit 1982), and age at marriage. All the above-mentioned studies highlighted the significance of these variables, thus making it imperative to include them in the analysis of the relationship of ethnicity and fertility.

However, there are a number of variables to be included in the analysis that had not been previously studied. In this study, variables like ethnic affiliation, ethnic fertility approval, woman's perceived role, and spouse interaction were also examined.

Theoretical Framework

The theoretical framework used in the study was developed by the five ASEAN country teams participating in the research project. The inter-relationships of all of the variables are expressed in terms of a path diagram which embraces all the hypotheses to be tested. Altogether there are three general models of analysis; one dealing with cumulative fertility (as measured by the number of children born to a woman during her reproductive period) as the dependent variable, another dealing with current contraceptive practice as the dependent variable, and the last treating recent fertility (as measured by the number of children born to a woman during the last 5 years) as the dependent variable. The three models involve a similar set of variables, differing only in the causal ordering of the independent variables and the dependent variable.

According to Model I, which is used to analyse cumulative fertility, it is hypothesized that age and the degree of wife's ethnic affiliation are negatively related to her education. Current age, a cohort variable, is expected to have a negative relationship with woman's age at first marriage. Woman's education, in turn, will be negatively related to husband's dominance, positively related to her employment and negatively related to her ethnic fertility approval and religiosity. Female employment will also be negatively related to husband's dominance and negatively related to child mortality experience and months of breastfeeding. Husband's dominance is expected to be positively related to son preference, which is, in turn, expected to affect positively desired family size and to relate negatively with contraceptive practice. The degree of religiosity and perceived woman's role are positively related to the psychic cost of contraceptive practice. Recent fertility, the second dependent variable, is set to be affected negatively by woman's age at first marriage, months of breastfeeding and contraception, and positively by desired family size.

Figure 1.1 differs from Figure 1.2 only in that it leaves out the current contraceptive practice on the basis that the dependent variable, cumulative fertility, includes all the events that occurred to a woman probably long before she practiced contraception. The rest of the model remains intact.

Figure 1.3 differs from Figure 1.1 in that it substitutes current contraceptive practice as the dependent variable for cumulative fertility. The rest of the diagram is the same as Figure 1.1.

However, it should be noted that even though the conceptual framework is expressed in terms of a path diagram, data analysis will not be restricted to the use of path analysis as the technique has some limitations or restrictive assumptions that other techniques such as multiple classification analysis and analysis of variance do not have.

The following chapter will present the methodology of the research project. It will describe the sampling design and its representativeness, the questionnaire, field procedures and an evaluation of data quality. This will be followed by an analysis of differences among the four ethnic groups in social, economic and demographic characteristics; then an analysis of ethnic

FIGURE 1.1

Path Model of Ethnicity, Socio-Economic Variables, and Cumulative Fertility

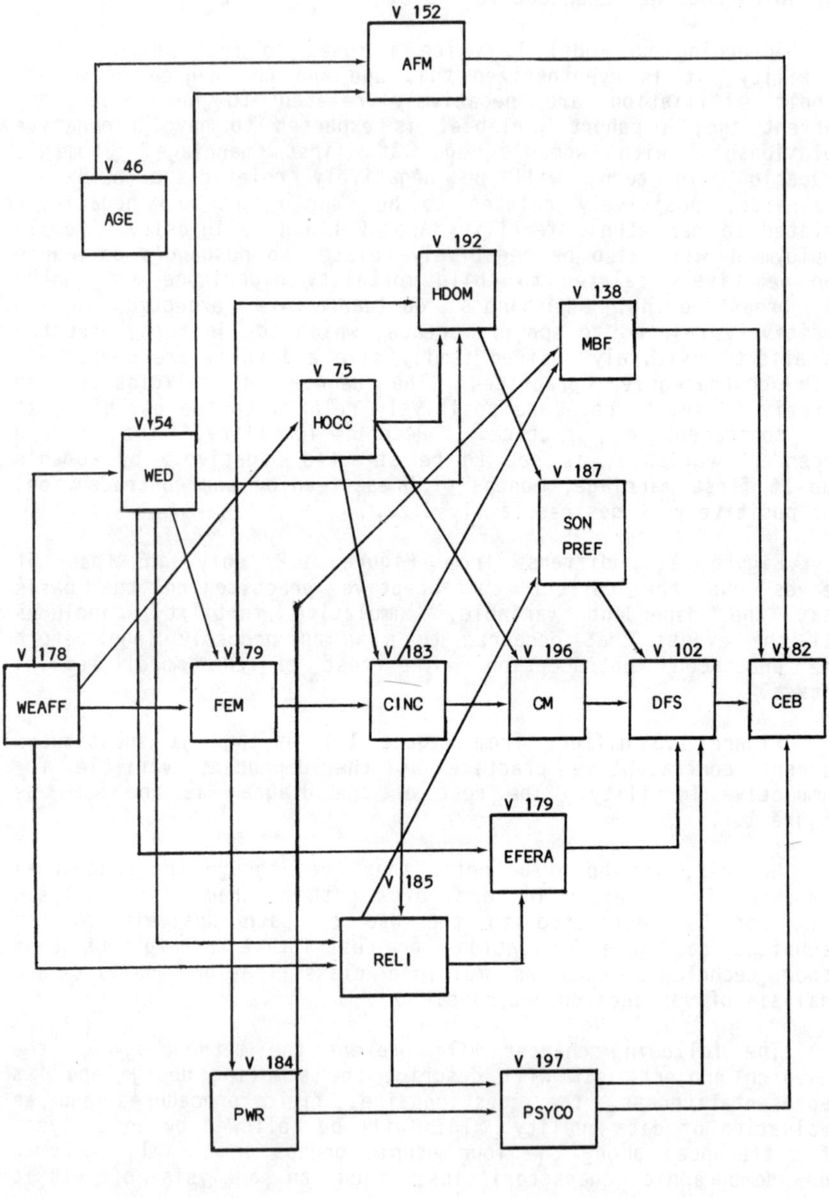

NOTE: For Abbreviations of Variables, see Appendix A.

FIGURE 1.2
Path Model of Ethnicity, Socio-Economic Variables, and Recent Fertility

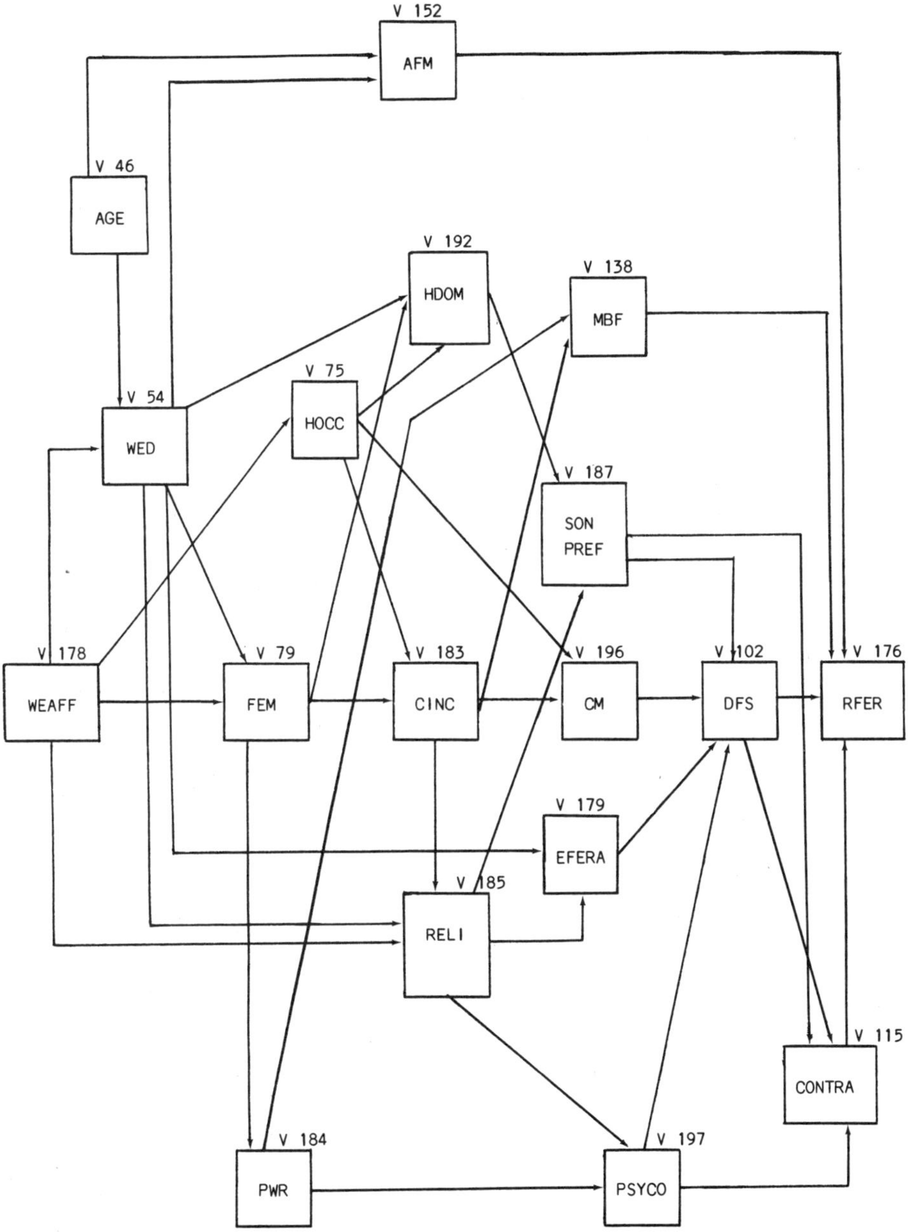

NOTE: For Abbreviations of Variables, see Appendix A.

FIGURE 1.3
Path Model of Ethnicity, Socio-Economic Variables, and Contraception

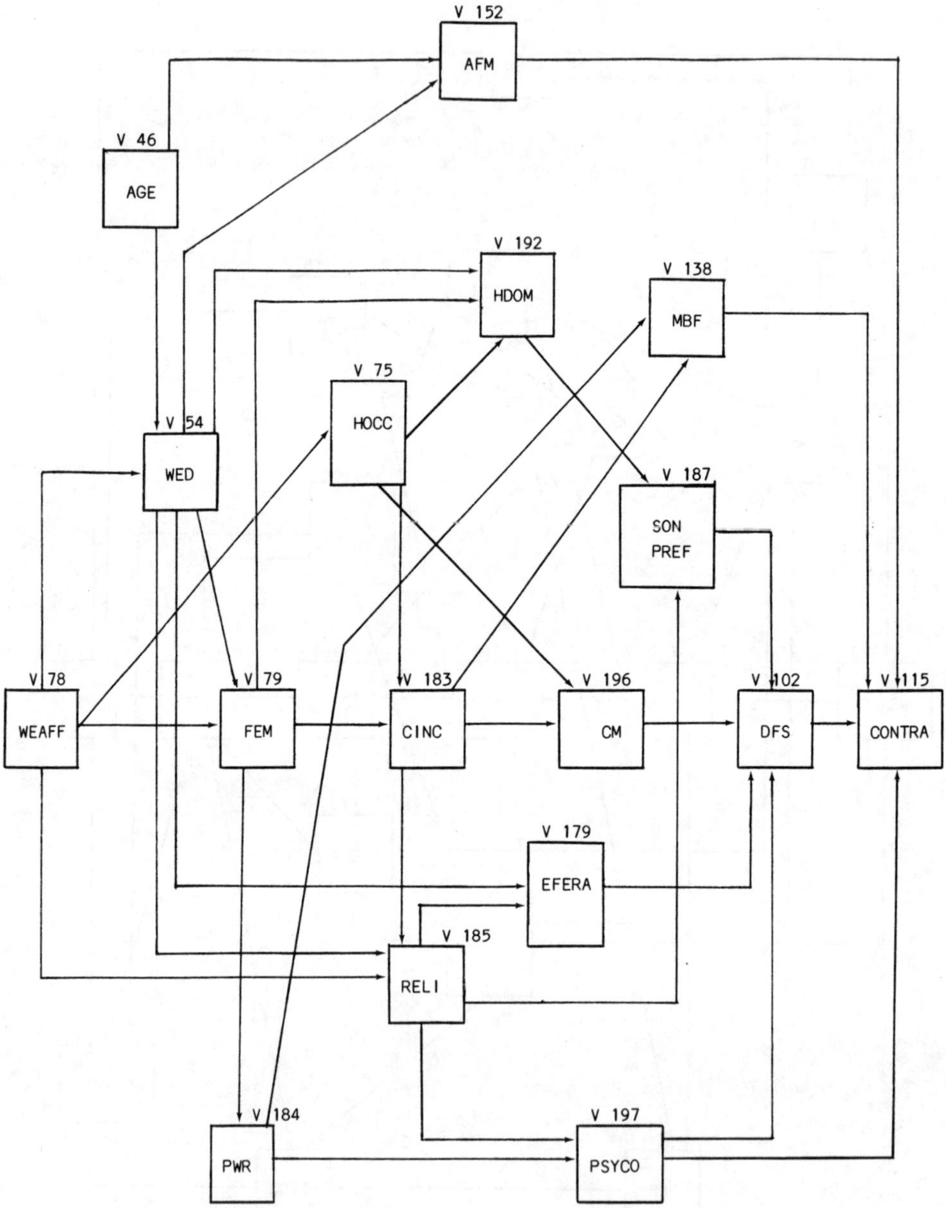

NOTE: For Abbreviations of Variables, see Appendix A.

differences in fertility and other fertility related measures. An attempt will be made to explain ethnic differences in fertility with the use of various multiple-variate techniques including MCA, ANOVA, multiple regression and path analysis. Finally, a summary of findings, limitations of the study and further desirable research and theoretical and practical implications, will be presented.

II

RESEARCH METHODOLOGY

The research project is based on a sample survey of all four major regions of the country. Map 2.1 shows the geographical division of the country and the distribution of the areas covered by the research project. A major methodological difficulty in studying the issues of ethnicity and fertility is the distribution of the ethnic groups. On the whole the various ethnic groups, by culture and preference, seem to congregate in certain areas.

In Thailand, the great majority of the Thai Muslims concentrate in four Southern provinces where they form the majority of the provincial population. The rest of the Thai Muslims are scattered throughout the country. For instance, in some Northeastern provinces, one will find pockets of Thai Muslims living in communities where they constitute a minority population. The great majority of Chinese live in urban areas. Only in very large provinces can one find some Chinese living in rural areas. Further complicating the sampling procedure is the fact that there are significant differences among the four major regions and between urban and rural areas. To carry out the research project, a special sampling design was called for.

Target Population and Sampling Design

Target Population

The target population of the research project includes four major groups of people: the Thais, the Chinese, the Southern Thai Muslims and the Thai Muslims. The last two groups require

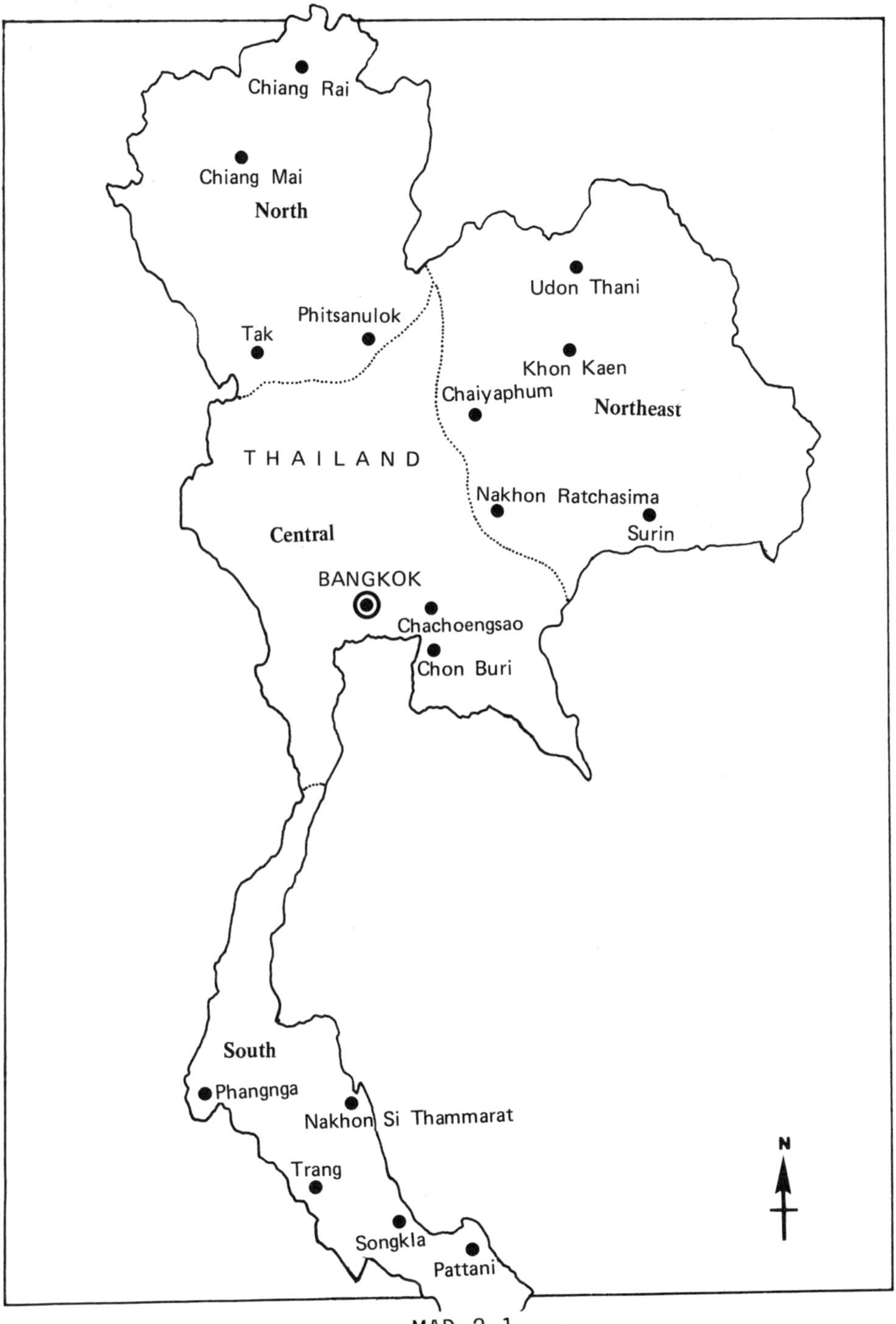

MAP 2.1
Distribution of Sample

some comment. The Southern Thai Muslims are predominantly Thai Muslims, constituting about 60 per cent of all Thai Muslims, and live mostly in the four southernmost provinces of Thailand. Other Thai Muslims are not, strictly speaking, a homogenous ethnic group, since they include Pakistanis, Yunnanese, and others. Non-Malay Thai Muslims are scattered throughout the country, so that it is possible to make comparisons between them and the Thai and Chinese who live in various regions of Thailand. Little is known about how Thai Muslim fertility differs from the Southern Thai Muslim fertility, which is an additional reason for studying both groups. It would be preferable to study a specific group among the non-Southern Thai Muslims, but this is precluded by the small size of each of these groups.

The sampling procedure began with the stratification of the population by region. The provinces in each region were then sampled in proportion to the size of the population. In each sampled province, a municipal area constituted an urban area, and a non-municipal area, a rural area. The sampling procedure posed no problem to the sample of Thai and urban Chinese but it did in the sample of rural Chinese and Thai Muslims, who constituted very small minorities in some of the sampled provinces. As the field survey in each region was conducted by a regional team, the regional co-investigators were allowed to include all the Chinese and the Thai Muslims found in the communities. If the number was still inadequate, they could find an additional number from the nearest community, district, or province until they obtained the desired number of cases.

For the Muslims, once the provinces were sampled, the concentrations of the ethnic groups in the rural areas were then identified, pre-surveyed and sampled. Contact was made with religious leaders and caretakers of the mosques for the lists of the Muslim members of the communities. The co-operation of community leaders was also solicited. Eligible persons were later identified and sampled.

All the urban or municipal areas of the sampled provinces were surveyed. Contact was made with local officials to inform them of the nature of the research and to get their assistance in identifying communities of the target groups. These communities were then sampled in proportion to the size.

The households in the sampled communities or areas were listed and systematically sampled. Replacements were allowed when the household heads refused to be interviewed. In such cases, the interviewers were instructed to go to the nearest household to reach the required number.

Eligibility for interview was based on the following

criteria for males. He must be a member of one of the ethnic groups, currently married and a major income earner of the household. For females, she must be currently married and aged between 15 and 44. Both husband and wife should be from the same ethnic group and must be living together.

It was proposed that the total sample size include 2,000 wives and 800 husbands. The proposed distribution of the sample is shown in Table 2.1. In actuality, the total sample size includes 2,237 wives and 841 husbands, exceeding the proposed sample size by 278 cases.

Table 2.2 shows the distribution of the sample by ethnic group, by region, province and by urban/rural residence.

Questionnaire and Field Procedures

The questionnaire used in the survey is the core questionnaire developed by the researchers of the five participating countries through a series of workshops. The questionnaire was translated from English into Thai and then translated back from Thai into English by the principal investigator and his research team in Bangkok. No pre-testing of the final questionnaire was done, as all the questions included had to be asked in the way that all the countries had agreed upon, and the pre-test of the earlier versions of the questionnaire had already been conducted.

The field-work was conducted by four regional teams: the Northern, the Central, the Northeastern and the Southern. All regional teams were led by senior faculty members of the major regional universities. The Northern team was led by Mr Luechai Chulasai of the Department of Economics, Chiangmai University. Some of his research team members came from the Department of Sociology and Anthropology. The Southern team was led by Ms Saranya Bunnag of the Faculty of Management Science, Prince of Songkla University. The Northeastern team was led by Mr Tawatchai Arthornthurasook, Faculty of Social Sciences and Humanities, Mahidol University. The Central team was co-led by Mr Suchart Prasithrathsint and Ms Suwanlee Piampiti, both of the School of Applied Statistics, National Institute of Development Administration.

A meeting was held of the leaders of the regional teams to reach agreement on the scope and areas of responsibility. Each regional team had complete control over the field research activities and use of data. However, general guidelines on the ethnic and sex composition of the interviewers, sampling

TABLE 2.1

Distribution by Ethnic Group, Urban-Rural Residence, and Sex

Area	Total Actual Sample Size	Thai				Chinese				Southern Thai Muslim				Thai Muslim			
		Wives		Husbands		Wives		Husbands		Wives		Husbands		Wives		Husbands	
		P	A	P	A	P	A	P	A	P	A	P	A	P	A	P	A
Urban																	
North	296	75	77	25	25	75	80	25	29	-	-	-	-	75	64	25	21
Northeast	320	75	80	25	28	75	80	25	28	-	-	-	-	75	76	25	28
Central	275	75	76	25	26	75	76	25	26	-	-	-	-	75	53	25	18
South	667	75	94	25	28	75	76	25	30	200	214	100	108	75	83	25	34
Subtotal	1,558	300	327	100	107	300	312	100	113	200	214	100	108	300	276	100	101
Rural																	
North	288	75	83	25	27	75	75	25	27	-	-	-	-	75	49	25	27
Northeast	286	75	81	25	28	75	79	25	27	-	-	-	-	75	51	25	20
Central	312	75	76	25	26	75	76	25	26	-	-	-	-	75	80	25	28
South	634	75	88	25	31	75	77	25	28	200	200	100	106	75	78	25	26
Subtotal	1,520	300	328	100	112	300	307	100	108	200	200	100	106	300	258	100	101
Total	3,078	600	655	200	219	600	619	200	221	400	414	200	214	600	534	200	202

NOTE: P = proposed sample size; A = actual sample size.

procedures and other administrative matters were discussed, agreed upon and followed.

Each team of 14 consisted of 7 pairs of male and female interviewers. They were composed of students, faculty members of the regional universities, and public school teachers in the respective regions. The interviewers were selected on the basis of (1) experience in interviewing, (2) ability to speak the local dialect and Chinese, and (3) being a member of an ethnic group.

The recruits were given sets of the questionnaire and an interviewer's guide to study prior to training sessions. They were given two days' training before starting the field survey. Field practice was conducted to help improve their skill and test their interviewing abilities. After the field practice, a meeting was held to discuss problematic questions and other general problems associated with locating and identifying respondents.

The selected locations were first surveyed by the regional co-investigators, public school teachers, and field supervisors. They pre-listed and mapped the households that qualified as respondents in terms of wife's age, husband's presence and spouses' ethnicity. Out of each list, potential respondents were systematically sampled.

There were no problems in locating Thai respondents in rural and urban areas as they comprised the majority of the Thai people. They were pre-listed and sampled by the regional team leaders and supervisors during the preliminary field surveys. For the Chinese ethnic group in the urban areas, the problem was not locating them but getting their co-operation in granting interviews. This problem occurred even in the pre-listing stage. In the rural areas there were very few Chinese and this posed a problem. Many of them also denied their Chinese origins while others could not differentiate ethnicity from nationality and were adamant that they were Thai. The Thai Muslims, except in the South, were also scattered and few in numbers. The problem was more severe in rural areas in other regions than in the South and in urban areas.

Three sources of help in locating respondents were:

(a) the recruited students and their relatives who lived in the selected areas,

(b) heads or caretakers of the mosques who keep updated lists of the mosque members, and

TABLE 2.2

Distribution of Sample by Ethnic Group, Residence, and Region

Ethnicity	Region	Province	Residence	Couples	Wives
THAI	Central	Bangkok	Urban	10	20
			Rural	10	20
		Chon Buri	Urban	7	14
			Rural	7	14
		Chachoengsao	Urban	8	16
			Rural	8	16
	Northeast	Nakorn Ratch-sima	Urban	9	18
			Rural	9	17
		Khon Kaen	Urban	9	17
			Rural	9	17
		Udonthani	Urban	-	-
			Rural	9	19
		Chaiyaphum	Urban	5	10
			Rural	-	-
		Surin	Urban	4	7
			Rural	-	-
	North	Chiangrai	Urban	-	-
			Rural	18	38
		Chiangmai	Urban	8	16
			Rural	-	-
		Phitsanulok	Urban	8	18
			Rural	-	-
		Tak	Urban	8	18
			Rural	8	18
	South	Nakhon Si-Thammarat	Urban	8	22
			Rural	19	43
		Songkla	Urban	13	26
			Rural	-	-
		Trang	Urban	6	18
			Rural	-	-
		Phangnga	Urban	-	-
			Rural	2	4
		Pattani	Urban	-	-
			Rural	9	10

TABLE 2.2 (cont'd)
Distribution of Sample by Ethnic Group, Residence, and Region

Ethnicity	Region	Province	Residence	Couples	Wives
		Bangkok	Urban	10	20
			Rural	10	20
	Central	Chon Buri	Urban	7	14
			Rural	8	22
		Chachoengsao	Urban	8	16
			Rural	7	8
		Nakhon Ratch-	Urban	9	18
		sima	Rural	8	18
		Khon Kaen	Urban	9	17
			Rural	9	17
	Northeast				
		Udonthani	Urban	-	-
			Rural	9	17
		Chaiyaphum	Urban	9	17
CHINESE		& Surin	Rural	-	-
		Chiangrai	Urban	28	51
	North	Chiangmai			
		Tak & Phit-			
		sanulok	Rural	26	48
		Nakhon Si-	Urban	9	13
		Thammarat	Rural	17	33
		Songkla	Urban	13	25
			Rural	-	-
		Trang	Urban	7	8
			Rural	-	-
		Phangnga	Urban	-	-
			Rural	2	6
		Pattani	Urban	-	-
			Rural	8	10

TABLE 2.2 (cont'd)

Ethnicity	Region	Province	Residence	Couples	Wives
THAI MUSLIM	Central	Bangkok	Urban	10	20
			Rural	10	20
		Chon Buri	Urban	7	15
			Rural	8	16
	Northeast	Nakhon Ratch-sima	Rural	9	16
		Khon Kaen	Urban	9	16
			Rural	7	16
		Udonthani	Urban	9	11
		Ubon Ratch-thani	Urban	-	14
		Chaiyaphum	Urban	-	2
		Si Sa Ket	Urban	7	3
		Surin	Urban	2	2
		Udonthani & Surin	Rural	10	15
	North	Chiangmai Chiangrai	Urban	20	43
		Tak & Phit-sanulok	Rural	26	22
	South	Nakhon Si-Thammarat	Urban	12	17
			Rural	17	35
		Songkla	Urban	13	25
		Trang	Urban	8	7
		Pattani	Rural	6	13
		Phangnga	Rural	2	4
SOUTHERN THAI MUSLIM	South	Pattani	Urban	55	57
			Rural	52	47
		Yala	Urban	51	49
			Rural	52	47
	TOTAL			841	1,396

(c) community leaders, such as village headmen and local authorities.

With respect to field supervision, each regional team had its own supervisors. In all cases, they were the regional co-investigators and their research associates and assistants. The questionnaires were checked on the spot after the interviews. Incomplete and doubtful questionnaires were returned to the interviewers to be verified with the interviewees. After each day's work, the field supervisors re-checked the questionnaires again before leaving the survey areas and appropriate action was taken as problems arose.

On the average, each interview took 45 minutes for a female respondent and 30 minutes a male respondent.

In general, efforts were made to match the interviewers and the respondents by sex, language or dialect, and ethnicity. However, female interviewers were more frequently used to interview male respondents as it was more socially and culturally acceptable than using male interviewers to interview female respondents on private matters such as contraceptive practices.

Generally, the rural respondents were more co-operative than their urban counterparts. Quite a number of the urban people flatly refused to be interviewed. Among the three ethnic groups, the Thais and Thai Muslims were more co-operative than the Chinese. The Chinese seemed to be fearful that the information given might have detrimental effects on their security.

Insofar as data processing is concerned, the country codebook is based on the categorization of the responses given by the inter-country co-ordinator. Attempts were made to follow categorical codes as much as possible. In many cases, a one-column code was used instead of a two-column code as dictated by the factual responses.

The coding of all the interview schedules was done in Bangkok by experienced coders who had been involved in a number of research projects previously. They tried the coding instructions, noted difficult and questionable codes, and standardized the codes after consulting with a coding supervisor and the principal investigator.

A close examination of the quality of data based on frequency distributions and detailed cross-tabulations of a number of variables, unquestionably reveals that the data collected and processed are of the best that could be obtained in a national sample survey.

III

THE NATURE OF ETHNIC DIFFERENCES

Even though the problems of minorities have long attracted the attention of Thai scholars, policy-makers and the general public, no solid empirical evidence has been gathered to contrast and compare their demographic, socio-economic and ethnic differences. Data collected by the researcher provided, for the first time, a great opportunity to study empirically the differences among the four major ethnic groups in Thailand, namely Thais, Chinese, Thai Muslims and Southern Thai Muslims. The first part contrasts the ethnic characteristics of the four ethnic groups while the second part highlights their demographic and socio-economic differences.

Contrasts of Ethnic Characteristics of Ethnic Groups

Parental Ethnicity

The great majority of the respondents have the same ethnicity as their parents. Over 90 per cent of the respondents have fathers of their own ethnic stock, and no less than three-fourths have mothers belonging to the same ethnic groups (Table 3.1). It is interesting to note that about one-fourth of the Chinese respondents have Thai mothers; about 2 per cent of the Thais have Chinese mothers; more than 10 percent of the Thai Muslims have Thai mothers; and about 4 per cent of the Southern Thai Muslims have Thai Muslim mothers. This would indicate that the Chinese and the Thai Muslims in various parts of the country are more liberal towards inter-ethnic marraiges than the Thais and the Southern Thai Muslims.

Birthplace

In general, over half of the respondents were born in their respective home regions. However, there are some variations by ethnic groups. More Chinese, who tend to be more mobile, were born outside their home regions. Next come the Thai Muslims and the Southern Thai Muslims. They were born probably in the country birthplace of their parents. The Thai respondents who stated they were born outside the home region simply reflects the rate of internal migration among this ethnic group (Table 3.2).

Citizenship

The overwhelming majority of the members of each ethnic group claimed Thai citizenship. Only a small percentage of the Chinese respondents claimed they were citizens of a foreign country, most probably mainland China.

Ethnic Identification

When asked to specify their ethnic identification the respondents exhibited a very strong ethnic identification with their own group. Over 90 per cent of the respondents of all ethnic groups always considered themselves members of their respective ethnic groups. About 7.2 per cent of the Chinese women and 9 per cent of the Chinese men sometimes considered themselves members of other ethnic groups, most probably Thai. Among the Thai Muslims, only 3.5 per cent of the women and a slightly higher percentage of the men sometimes considered themselves something other than a member of their own ethnic group. Here again they probably considered themselves Thai.

Ethnic versus National Identification

Regarding the relative importance of ethnic versus national identification, the female members of the Thai, the Thai Muslim and the Southern Thai Muslim stress the significance of ethnic over national identification while the male members of all ethnic groups and Chinese women consider both ethnic and national identification equally important.

TABLE 3.1

Percentage of Respondents by Ethnic Group

Variable	Chinese				Thai			
	Rural		Urban		Rural		Urban	
	Female	Male	Female	Male	Female	Male	Female	Male
Father's Ethnicity								
Chinese	98.4	98.1	99.7	100.0	2.5	1.8	2.5	5.0
Indian	-	-	-	-	-	-	-	-
Maranao	-	-	-	-	0.3	-	-	-
Thai	1.6	1.9	0.3	-	97.2	98.2	97.0	95.0
Thai Muslim	-	-	-	-	-	-	-	-
Southern Thai Muslims	-	-	-	-	-	-	-	-
Pakistani	-	-	-	-	-	-	-	-
Caucasian	-	-	-	-	-	-	-	-
Total	100.0	100.0	100.0	100.0	100.0	100.0	100.0	100.0

TABLE 3.1 (cont'd)

Variable	Thai Muslim				Southern Thai Muslim			
	Rural		Urban		Rural		Urban	
	Female	Male	Female	Male	Female	Male	Female	Male
Father's Ethnicity								
Chinese	0.7	1.8	1.6	0.9	-	-	-	-
Indian	-	-	0.6	2.7	-	1.0	-	-
Maranao	-	-	0.3	-	-	-	-	-
Thai	2.7	1.8	0.9	1.8	-	1.0	0.6	-
Thai Muslim	88.9	92.0	93.7	91.9	3.0	5.0	2.6	5.2
Southern Thai Muslims	5.4	-	-	-	97.0	93.0	95.8	92.7
Pakistani	2.3	4.4	2.5	2.7	-	-	1.0	2.1
Caucasian	-	-	0.4	-	-	-	-	-
Total	100.0	100.0	100.0	100.0	100.0	100.0	100.0	100.0

TABLE 3.1 (cont'd)
Percentage of Respondents by Ethnic Group

Variable	Chinese				Thai			
	Rural		Urban		Rural		Urban	
	Female	Male	Female	Male	Female	Male	Female	Male
Mother's Ethnicity								
Chinese	75.9	77.6	78.6	86.5	1.2	1.8	0.9	3.0
Indian	-	-	-	-	-	-	-	-
Thai	24.1	22.4	20.8	13.5	98.8	98.2	98.8	96.0
Thai Muslim	-	-	0.3	-	-	-	-	-
Southern Thai Muslims	-	-	0.3	-	-	-	-	-
Lao	-	-	-	-	-	-	0.3	-
Pakistani	-	-	-	-	-	-	-	-
Burmese	-	-	-	-	-	-	-	1.0
Total	100.0	100.0	100.0	100.0	100.0	100.0	100.0	100.0

TABLE 3.1 (cont'd)

Variable	Thai Muslim				Southern Thai Muslim			
	Rural		Urban		Rural		Urban	
	Female	Male	Female	Male	Female	Male	Female	Male
Mother's Ethnicity								
Chinese	0.3	-	0.3	-	-	-	-	-
Indian	-	-	-	0.9	-	-	-	-
Thai	10.5	11.6	12.4	14.4	-	3.0	-	-
Thai Muslim	83.5	86.6	86.1	83.8	3.0	5.9	5.2	8.3
Southern Thai Muslims	5.1	-	-	-	97.0	91.1	94.8	91.7
Lao	0.3	0.9	-	-	-	-	-	-
Pakistani	0.3	0.9	0.9	0.9	-	-	-	-
Burmese	-	-	0.3	-	-	-	-	-
Total	100.0	100.0	100.0	100.0	100.0	100.0	100.0	100.0

TABLE 3.2
Birthplace, Citizenship, Ethnic Identification and
Ethnic versus National Identification by Ethnic Groups

	Chinese				Thai			
	Rural		Urban		Rural		Urban	
Variable	Female	Male	Female	Male	Female	Male	Female	Male
Birthplace								
Home region	59.0	57.9	50.0	61.5	70.3	65.5	57.0	52.0
Neutral area	0.3	-	-	-	0.6	2.7	-	1.0
Other group's region	40.7	42.1	50.0	38.5	29.1	31.8	43.0	47.0
Total	100.0	100.0	100.0	100.0	100.0	100.0	100.0	100.0
Citizenship								
Other country	3.6	3.7	0.3	1.0	0.3	-	-	-
This country	96.4	96.3	99.7	99.0	99.7	100.0	100.0	100.0
Total	100.0	100.0	100.0	100.0	100.0	100.0	100.0	100.0
Ethnic identification								
Always considers self group member	92.5	89.7	92.8	91.4	99.7	100.0	100.0	100.0
Sometimes something else	7.5	10.3	7.2	8.6	0.3	-	-	-
Total	100.0	100.0	100.0	100.0	100.0	100.0	100.0	100.0
Ethnic versus National identification (per cent)								
Ethnic more important	20.6	34.3	20.6	21.7	46.4	17.6	48.4	20.0
Equally important	47.5	46.7	49.7	42.5	38.1	40.0	31.4	33.8
Nationality more important	32.4	19.0	29.7	35.8	15.5	42.0	19.9	46.4
Not citizen	-	-	-	-	-	-	0.3	-
Total	100.0	100.0	100.0	100.0	100.0	100.0	100.0	100.0

TABLE 3.2 (cont'd)

Variable	Thai Muslim				Southern Thai Muslim			
	Rural		Urban		Rural		Urban	
	Female	Male	Female	Male	Female	Male	Female	Male
Birthplace								
Home region	62.0	57.1	64.2	63.1	69.0	60.4	61.7	51.0
Neutral area	-	-	-	0.9	-	-	-	-
Other group's region	38.0	42.9	35.8	36.0	31.0	39.6	38.3	49.0
Total	100.0	100.0	100.0	100.0	100.0	100.0	100.0	100.0
Citizenship								
Other country	0.3	0.9	0.6	0.9	-	1.0	-	-
This country	99.7	99.1	99.4	99.1	100.0	99.0	100.0	100.0
Total	100.0	100.0	100.0	100.0	100.0	100.0	100.0	100.0
Ethnic identification								
Always considers self group member	96.6	96.4	95.3	91.9	98.5	100.0	97.9	99.0
Sometimes something else	3.4	3.6	4.7	8.1	1.5	-	2.1	1.0
Total	100.0	100.0	100.0	100.0	100.0	100.0	100.0	100.0
Ethnic versus National identification (per cent)								
Ethnic more important	44.7	17.1	39.1	22.3	40.6	7.4	41.8	5.0
Equally important	34.6	36.9	45.8	43.8	52.6	51.8	51.0	45.5
Nationality more important	20.1	45.9	14.8	33.9	6.8	41.1	7.1	49.5
Not citizen	0.2	-	0.3	-	0.0	-	0.0	-
Total	100.0	100.0	100.0	100.0	100.0	100.0	100.0	100.0

Language

Mother Tongue

Except for the Southern Thai Muslims, Thai is the mother tongue of the great majority of the Thais, the Chinese and the Thai Muslims (Table 3.3). The mother tongue of the Southern Thai Muslims is Malay. However, about 15 per cent of the Chinese used Chinese as their mother tongue; less than one per cent of the Thai used Khmer, Burmese or Lao as their mother tongue; about 5 per cent of the Thai Muslims use Malay as their mother tongue; and 6 per cent of the Southern Thai Muslims use Thai as their mother tongue.

Language Used at Home

As for the language most commonly spoken at home, the great majority of the respondents speak Thai, except the Southern Thai Muslim. More than 90 per cent of the Southern Thai Muslim continue to use Malay as their home language. The percentage variation in language spoken at home implies the degree of assimilation of the members of ethnic groups into the Thai society.

Language Used with Friends and at Work

Thai is also the major language spoken with friends and at work by the great majority of the respondents, again with the exception of the Southern Thai Muslims. It is interesting to note that among the Chinese, the percentage of Chinese used with friends and at work is lower than that of its usage at home. Normally, the Chinese have a mixed group of Thai and Chinese friends; under these circumstances, it is better for them to speak Thai than Chinese, unlike when they are in their home environs.

Language Preference

The majority of the Chinese (80 per cent), the Thai (85 per cent), and the Thai Muslims (81 per cent) prefer Thai language TV and radio programmes. The Southern Thai Muslim, however, are split over their language of preference. The percentage of those who prefer Malay language TV and radio programmes is less than that of those who prefer Thai. Only a minority of the respondents of all ethnic groups expressed no language preference.

Regarding preference for language of newspapers, the majority of the members of all ethnic groups, including the Southern Thai Muslims, prefer to read Thai newspapers. This, to a considerable extent, reflects the success of the Thai educational system in providing basic primary education to its population compared with the failure of the TV programmes in capturing the attention of the Southern ethnic group.

Media Usage

About 60 per cent of the Chinese and 70 per cent the Southern Thai Muslims compared with less than half of the Thai and the Thai Muslims watch television regularly, probably reflecting the poorer economic conditions of the Thai and the Thai Muslims in general. As a result, they compensate by listening to radio more regularly than the Chinese. It is interesting to note that the majority of the Southern Thai Muslims also listen to radio regularly since TV programmes do not normally begin until fairly late in the evening.

The newspaper is read every day by half of the Chinese population. A lower percentage of the Thais read newspapers every day, followed by the Thai Muslims and the Southern Thai Muslims (Table 3.4). The percentage of those who never read newspapers is highest among the Southern Thai Muslims (about 55 per cent of the wives and 45 per cent of the husbands), followed by the Thai Muslims, the Thais and the Chinese. Husbands of all ethnic groups invariably show a higher percentage of newspaper readership than wives.

Religion and Religiosity

The overwhelming majority of the Thais and Chinese are Buddhist, and most of the Thai Muslims and the Southern Thai Muslims are followers of the Islamic faith. Religiosity as measured by the reported frequency of prayer and attendance at religious services is highest among the Southern Thai Muslims, followed by the Thai Muslims, the Thais and the Chinese respectivley; 80 per cent or more of the Southern Thai Muslims report they prayed several times a day compared with 49 per cent or more of the Thai Muslims and 5 per cent of the Thai and 3 per cent of the Chinese (Table

TABLE 3.3
Mother Tongue, Language Used at Home and at Work,
Language Used with Friends, and Language Preference by Ethnic Group

	Chinese				Thai			
	Rural		Urban		Rural		Urban	
Variable	Female	Male	Female	Male	Female	Male	Female	Male
Mother Tongue								
Chinese	14.3	12.1	16.7	17.1	-	-	-	-
Malay	-	-	-	-	-	-	-	-
Thai	85.4	87.9	82.1	81.9	99.1	100.0	100.0	99.0
Thai Muslim	-	-	0.3	-	-	-	-	-
English	-	-	0.3	1.0	-	-	-	-
Other	-	-	0.3	-	-	-	-	-
Khmer, Burmese, Laotian	0.3	-	0.3	-	0.9	-	-	1.0
Total	100.0	100.0	100.0	100.0	100.0	100.0	100.0	100.0
Language Used at Home								
Chinese	15.6	15.9	11.6	8.6	-	-	-	-
Malay	-	-	-	-	-	-	-	-
Thai	84.4	84.1	88.4	91.4	99.1	100.0	99.7	99.0
Thai Muslim	-	-	-	-	-	-	-	-
Other	-	-	-	-	-	-	-	-
Khmer, Burmese, Laotian	-	-	-	-	0.9	-	-	1.0
Laos	-	-	-	-	-	-	0.3	-
Total	100.0	100.0	100.0	100.0	100.0	100.0	100.0	100.0
Language Used with Friends								
Chinese	11.1	9.3	4.1	11.4	-	-	-	-
Malay	-	-	-	-	-	-	-	-
Thai	88.9	90.7	95.9	88.6	98.8	100.0	99.4	100.0
Thai Muslim	-	-	-	-	-	-	-	-
Other	-	-	-	-	0.3	-	-	-
Khmer, Burmese, Lao	-	-	-	-	0.9	-	0.3	-
Laos	-	-	-	-	-	-	0.3	-
Total	100.0	100.0	100.0	100.0	100.0	100.0	100.0	100.0

TABLE 3.3 (cont'd)

Variable	Thai Muslim				Southern Thai Muslim			
	Rural		Urban		Rural		Urban	
	Female	Male	Female	Male	Female	Male	Female	Male
Mother Tongue								
Chinese	-	-	-	-	-	-	-	-
Malay	5.7	0.9	5.0	9.9	95.4	93.1	89.0	94.7
Thai	91.3	98.2	93.8	89.2	4.1	6.9	8.9	3.2
Thai Muslim	3.0	0.9	0.3	-	-	-	-	-
English	-	-	-	-	-	-	-	-
Other	-	-	-	0.9	0.5	-	2.1	2.1
Khmer, Burmese, Laotian	-	-	0.9	-	-	-	-	-
Total	100.0	100.0	100.0	100.0	100.0	100.0	100.0	100.0
Language Used at Home								
Chinese	-	-	0.3	-	-	-	-	-
Malay	5.4	0.9	5.7	10.8	96.9	98.0	93.2	93.7
Thai	91.9	99.1	93.4	89.2	2.1	1.0	5.2	4.2
Thai Muslim	2.7	-	-	-	-	-	-	-
Other	-	-	-	-	1.0	1.0	1.6	2.1
Khmer, Burmese, Laotian	-	-	0.6	-	-	-	-	-
Laos	-	-	-	-	-	-	-	-
Total	100.0	100.0	100.0	100.0	100.0	100.0	100.0	100.0
Language Used with Friends								
Chinese	-	-	-	-	-	-	-	-
Malay	6.1	1.8	4.1	10.0	92.2	93.8	83.5	87.4
Thai	91.5	98.2	95.3	90.0	6.8	5.2	14.4	9.5
Thai Muslim	2.4	-	-	-	-	-	-	-
Other	-	-	-	-	1.0	1.0	2.1	3.1
Khmer, Burmese, Lao	-	-	0.6	-	-	-	-	-
Laos	-	-	-	-	-	-	-	-
Total	100.0	100.0	100.0	100.0	100.0	100.0	100.0	100.0

TABLE 3.3 (cont'd)

Mother Tongue, Language Used at Home and at Work, Language Used with Friends, and Language Preference by Ethnic Group

Variable	Chinese				Thai			
	Rural		Urban		Rural		Urban	
	Female	Male	Female	Male	Female	Male	Female	Male
Language Used at Work								
Chinese	8.5	6.0	2.6	3.3	-	-	-	-
Malay	-	-	-	-	-	-	-	-
Thai	91.5	94.0	97.4	96.7	99.5	100.0	100.0	100.0
Thai Muslim	-	-	-	-	-	-	-	-
English	-	-	-	-	-	-	-	-
Other	-	-	-	-	-	-	-	-
Khmer, Burmese, Laotian	-	-	-	-	0.5	-	-	-
Total	100.0	100.0	100.0	100.0	100.0	100.0	100.0	100.0
Language Preferred for Radio or TV Programs								
Chinese	3.9	7.5	1.6	2.9	0.3	-	-	-
Malay	-	-	-	-	-	-	-	-
Thai	78.2	80.4	82.5	80.8	83.3	87.2	88.2	91.1
Thai Muslim	-	-	-	-	-	-	-	-
English	-	0.9	-	1.0	0.3	0.9	-	-
Other	0.3	-	-	-	-	-	-	-
No preference	17.6	11.2	15.9	15.3	16.1	11.9	11.8	8.9
Total	100.0	100.0	100.0	100.0	100.0	100.0	100.0	100.0
Languages of Newspapers Read								
Chinese	4.2	7.5	1.3	1.9	-	-	0.3	-
Malay	-	-	-	-	-	-	-	-
Thai	83.1	85.1	88.3	84.7	79.5	95.5	89.8	98.0
Thai and Chinese	1.6	3.7	0.3	1.9	-	-	-	-
No preference	11.1	3.7	9.8	9.6	20.5	3.6	9.9	2.0
Thai and English	-	-	0.3	1.9	-	0.9	-	-
Total	100.0	100.0	100.0	100.0	100.0	100.0	100.0	100.0

TABLE 3.3 (cont'd)

Variable	Thai Muslim				Southern Thai Muslim			
	Rural		Urban		Rural		Urban	
	Female	Male	Female	Male	Female	Male	Female	Male
Language Used at Work								
Chinese	-	-	-	-	-	-	-	-
Malay	2.1	1.9	4.9	6.2	85.4	75.0	67.4	64.2
Thai	96.4	96.3	93.2	92.8	13.6	25.0	32.6	35.8
Thai Muslim	1.5	0.9	0.5	-	-	-	-	-
English	-	-	-	1.0	-	-	-	-
Other	-	-	-	-	1.0	-	-	-
Khmer, Burmese, Laotian	-	0.9	1.4	-	-	-	-	-
Total	100.0	100.0	100.0	100.0	100.0	100.0	100.0	100.0
Language Preferred for Radio or TV Programs								
Chinese	-	-	-	-	-	-	-	-
Malay	7.1	2.7	2.2	7.2	44.7	40.0	42.5	40.0
Thai	81.4	79.5	82.9	86.5	46.7	55.0	48.7	53.7
Thai Muslim	1.7	-	0.3	-	-	-	-	-
English	-	0.8	-	0.9	-	-	-	-
Other	-	-	-	-	-	-	-	-
No preference	9.8	17.0	14.6	5.4	8.6	5.0	8.8	6.3
Total	100.0	100.0	100.0	100.0	100.0	100.0	100.0	100.0
Languages of Newspapers Read								
Chinese	-	-	-	-	-	-	-	-
Malay	-	-	-	-	-	1.9	-	1.7
Thai	76.5	89.2	87.7	94.6	66.4	90.7	84.1	98.3
Thai and Chinese	-	-	-	-	-	-	-	-
No preference	23.5	10.8	12.3	4.5	32.8	7.4	15.9	-
Thai and English	-	-	-	0.9	0.8	-	-	-
Total	100.0	100.0	100.0	100.0	100.0	100.0	100.0	100.0

TABLE 3.4
Mass Media Usage by Ethnic Group

Variable	Chinese				Thai			
	Rural		Urban		Rural		Urban	
	Female	Male	Female	Male	Female	Male	Female	Male
Per Cent Watching TV Regularly								
Yes	56.7	62.6	66.7	64.8	44.9	47.3	62.2	55.9
Per Cent Listening to Radio Regularly								
Yes	46.6	57.9	42.5	47.6	63.5	70.0	58.2	64.7
Frequency of Reading Newspaper								
Everyday	40.1	66.4	53.1	68.6	23.5	49.1	34.7	67.6
Several times a week	14.6	15.0	14.8	11.4	11.8	10.9	14.9	14.7
Once a week	3.3	2.8	3.5	1.9	7.4	11.9	5.9	2.0
Rarely	30.6	12.1	18.2	7.6	37.5	24.5	34.1	13.7
Never	11.4	3.7	10.4	10.5	19.8	3.6	10.4	2.0
Total	100.0	100.0	100.0	100.0	100.0	100.0	100.0	100.0

TABLE 3.4 (cont'd)

Variable	Thai Muslim				Southern Thai Muslim			
	Rural		Urban		Rural		Urban	
	Female	Male	Female	Male	Female	Male	Female	Male
Per Cent Watching TV Regularly								
Yes	40.7	46.4	59.7	61.3	72.1	77.2	65.8	69.5
Per Cent Listening to Radio Regularly								
Yes	51.9	64.3	51.6	58.6	81.7	87.1	67.9	71.6
Frequency of Reading Newspaper								
Everyday	18.9	38.4	37.4	62.2	9.6	19.8	10.4	22.3
Several times a week	13.9	23.2	17.6	10.8	3.6	5.0	6.2	10.6
Once a week	6.4	8.9	6.6	5.4	2.5	5.9	21.1	2.2
Rarely	36.8	18.8	25.8	17.1	25.4	19.8	26.4	28.7
Never	24.0	10.7	12.6	4.5	58.9	49.5	54.9	36.2
Total	100.0	100.0	100.0	100.0	100.0	100.0	100.0	100.0

3.5). The frequency of attendance at religious services of all ethnic groups further confirms that the Chinese and the Thais are less ceremonially religious than the Thai Muslims and the Southern Thai Muslims. Since, unlike Islam, there are no strict stipulations for attendance of religious services or frequency of prayer in Buddhism.

The overwhelming majority of the Southern Thai Muslims consider religion important in daily life. A lower percentage is found among the Thais, followed by the Muslims and the Chinese. The differences among the male and female members in this respect is almost non-existent.

Membership in Exclusive Ethnic Association

The great majority (over 80 per cent) of the members of all ethnic groups do not belong to any exclusive ethnic associations. Less than one-fourth the Chinese and the Thai Muslims belong to an exclusive ethnic association. The percentage of the Southern Thai Muslims who belong to an exclusive ethnic association is about 5 per cent, slightly less than the Thais. For all ethnic groups, the percentage of males who are members of exclusive associations is higher than that of females; and the rural percentage is higher than the urban one, except among the Thais. In the Thai sample, more urban than rural Thais belong to an ethnic association.

Ethnicity of Close Friends

Regarding ethnicity of close friends, the data clearly show that the Chinese and the Thai Muslims have close friends from their own ethnic groups as well as from other ethnic groups. However, the majority of the Thai and the Southern Thai Muslims (both form the majority in their own communities), claim that their close friends are members of their own ethnic groups. Thus, being a majority or a minority group in a community has an effect on the choice of close friends.

Ethnic Diversity Enriches a Nation's Culture

That ethnic diversity enriches a nation's culture is variably endorsed by different ethnic groups. The Chinese are most favourably disposed to the idea (as shown by a higher score), followed by the Thai Muslims, the Thai and the Southern Thai

Muslims (Table 3.6). The people in the rural areas are less liberal to the idea than their urban counterparts. The male Chinese, Thai Muslims and Southern Thai Muslims are more favourable to the idea than the females. The opposite is true among the Thais, implying Thai women are more conservative than Thai men in this regard.

Inter-Ethnic Marriage

Consistent with the findings on ethnic diversity and cultural enrichment, the Chinese and the Thai Muslims are more favourable towards inter-ethnic marriage than the Thai and the Southern Thai Muslims, respectively (as shown by a higher average score). Intermarriage is perceived less favourably by the female than the male members of all ethnic groups.

Relative Ease in Getting Ahead

On a group's relative ease in getting ahead these days as compared to other groups, the Chinese seem to be more optimistic as shown by higher scores than the Thai Muslims, the Thais and the Southern Thai Muslims, respectively. This is probably due to the fact that the Chinese and to some extent the Thai Muslims are engaged in commerce, industry, and cattle raising and a higher income than the other two groups, whose members are mostly engaged in lower income-earning activities in farming and wage earning.

Strength by Numbers

Responding to the statement that "an ethnic group can only be strong if there are many of them", a greater percentage of the Thai Muslims accept the statement as true compared with the Thais, the Southern Thai Muslims, and the Chinese respectively. A greater percentage of females also agree with the statement than their male counterparts, implying women are still more conservative in this regard than men.

When asked whether the socio-economic position of an ethnic group is better with many or few children, the majority of the respondents from all ethnic groups state that fewer children would be better. There are however ethnic differences: More Thais express their preference for few children than the Chinese, the Thai Muslims and the Southern Thai Muslims, respectively.

TABLE 3.5
Religion and Religiosity and Ethnic Affiliation by Ethnic Group

Variable	Chinese				Thai			
	Rural		Urban		Rural		Urban	
	Female	Male	Female	Male	Female	Male	Female	Male
Religion								
Islam	-	-	3.5	-	-	-	-	-
Protestant	1.3	0.9	1.3	3.8	0.6	0.9	0.6	-
Catholic	-	-	-	-	0.3	-	-	-
Buddhism	97.7	99.1	94.6	96.2	99.1	99.1	99.4	100.0
Ancestor worship	1.0	-	0.6	-	-	-	-	-
Total	100.0	100.0	100.0	100.0	100.0	100.0	100.0	100.0
Frequency of Prayer								
Never	25.1	30.8	36.1	34.3	14.9	9.1	13.9	14.7
Less than once a month	17.3	17.8	10.4	13.3	10.5	20.0	13.0	16.7
At least once a month	9.1	7.5	7.9	10.5	10.8	3.6	11.8	8.8
At least once a week	14.3	15.0	15.1	11.4	18.3	20.0	19.2	19.6
Once a day	31.6	25.2	26.7	26.7	39.6	41.8	39.0	36.3
Several times a day	2.6	3.7	3.8	3.8	5.9	5.5	3.1	3.9
Total	100.0	100.0	100.0	100.0	100.0	100.0	100.0	100.0

TABLE 3.5 (cont'd)

Variable	Thai Muslim				Southern Thai Muslim			
	Rural		Urban		Rural		Urban	
	Female	Male	Female	Male	Female	Male	Female	Male
Religion								
Islam	99.7	99.1	99.1	99.1	100.0	100.0	100.0	100.0
Protestant	-	-	-	-	-	-	-	-
Catholic	-	-	-	-	-	-	-	-
Buddhism	-	0.9	0.9	0.9	-	-	-	-
Ancestor worship	0.3	-	-	-	-	-	-	-
Total	100.0	100.0	100.0	100.0	100.0	100.0	100.0	100.0
Frequency of Prayer								
Never	15.5	5.3	13.9	7.2	1.6	1.0	0.5	1.1
Less than once a month	7.1	3.6	6.9	3.6	-	-	-	1.0
At least once a month	4.7	7.1	6.1	4.5	-	-	0.5	-
At least once a week	12.2	16.1	15.1	11.7	-	1.0	3.2	1.0
Once a day	12.2	13.4	15.1	19.8	8.6	15.8	8.8	2.1
Several times a day	48.3	54.5	42.9	53.2	89.8	82.2	87.0	94.8
Total	100.0	100.0	100.0	100.0	100.0	100.0	100.0	100.0

TABLE 3.5 (cont'd)
Religion and Religiosity and Ethnic Affiliation by Ethnic Group

Variable	Chinese				Thai			
	Rural		Urban		Rural		Urban	
	Female	Male	Female	Male	Female	Male	Female	Male
Attendance at Religious Services								
Never	16.8	19.6	19.2	23.7	11.8	7.3	10.2	18.6
Less than once a month	43.1	39.3	42.5	44.8	31.0	27.3	38.7	32.4
Once a month	16.3	12.1	16.4	8.6	23.2	20.9	18.6	15.7
Several times a month	17.0	16.8	8.2	8.6	16.7	20.9	17.6	17.6
Once a week	5.2	5.6	8.5	10.5	8.0	20.0	10.5	9.8
Several times a week	1.6	6.6	5.2	3.8	9.3	3.6	4.4	5.9
Total	100.0	100.0	100.0	100.0	100.0	100.0	100.0	100.0
Importance of Religion in Daily Life								
Not important	7.8	9.3	10.4	14.3	1.9	1.8	3.7	3.9
Quite important	89.6	89.7	88.4	81.9	97.2	98.2	95.4	96.1
Very important	2.6	1.0	1.2	3.8	0.9	-	0.9	-
Total	100.0	100.0	100.0	100.0	100.0	100.0	100.0	100.0

TABLE 3.5 (cont'd)

Variable	Thai Muslim				Southern Thai Muslim			
	Rural		Urban		Rural		Urban	
	Female	Male	Female	Male	Female	Male	Female	Male
Attendance at Religious Services								
Never	12.8	12.5	16.7	6.3	1.5	1.0	1.6	1.0
Less than once a month	29.4	16.2	30.3	17.2	-	-	4.1	-
Once a month	8.1	7.1	8.2	8.1	1.0	-	2.6	4.2
Several times a month	8.8	10.7	8.2	5.4	13.2	27.7	13.5	11.5
Once a week	26.4	44.6	21.5	43.2	10.7	16.8	12.4	15.6
Several times a week	14.5	8.9	15.1	19.8	73.6	54.5	65.8	67.7
Total	100.0	100.0	100.0	100.0	100.0	100.0	100.0	100.0
Importance of Religion in Daily Life								
Not important	2.4	1.8	1.9	1.8	0.5	-	-	-
Quite important	96.0	97.3	95.6	92.8	98.5	100.0	95.9	95.8
Very important	1.6	0.9	2.5	5.4	1.0	-	4.1	4.2
Total	100.0	100.0	100.0	100.0	100.0	100.0	100.0	100.0

TABLE 3.5 (cont'd)
Religion and Religiosity and Ethnic Affiliation by Ethnic Group

Variable	Chinese				Thai			
	Rural		Urban		Rural		Urban	
	Female	Male	Female	Male	Female	Male	Female	Male
Attendance at Ethnic or Religious Schools								
Attended own ethnic/ religious school	18.6	33.6	24.8	40.0	93.8	100.0	98.8	98.0
No schooling	6.8	4.7	5.7	2.9	6.2	-	1.2	1.0
Never attended own ethnic/religious school	74.6	61.7	69.5	57.1	-	-	-	1.0
Total	100.0	100.0	100.0	100.0	100.0	100.0	100.0	100.0
Membership in Exclusive Ethnic Associations								
Belong to own ethnic association	3.6	13.1	5.3	11.4	2.2	6.4	4.3	14.7
Do not belong to any association	93.5	75.7	88.4	69.5	94.1	85.4	93.2	74.5
Belong to other ethnic association	2.9	11.2	6.3	19.1	3.7	8.2	2.5	10.8
Total	100.0	100.0	100.0	100.0	100.0	100.0	100.0	100.0
Ethnicity of Close Friends								
All of own group	17.8	20.6	14.5	14.3	62.8	52.7	52.6	37.6
Some own group, some other	81.2	79.4	83.9	83.8	36.6	47.3	46.4	62.4
No close friends	1.0	-	1.6	1.9	0.6	-	1.0	-
Total	100.0	100.0	100.0	100.0	100.0	100.0	100.0	100.0

TABLE 3.5 (cont'd)

Variable	Thai Muslim				Southern Thai Muslim			
	Rural		Urban		Rural		Urban	
	Female	Male	Female	Male	Female	Male	Female	Male
Attendance at Ethnic or Religious Schools								
Attended own ethnic/ religious school	36.4	42.0	27.7	31.8	48.3	62.0	40.1	40.0
No schooling	7.1	5.4	7.2	0.9	22.3	9.0	30.2	17.9
Never attended own ethnic/religious school	56.5	52.6	65.1	67.3	29.4	29.0	29.7	42.1
Total	100.0	100.0	100.0	100.0	100.0	100.0	100.0	100.0
Membership in Exclusive Ethnic Associations								
Belong to own ethnic association	13.8	18.7	10.7	13.5	1.0	6.0	3.1	5.3
Do not belong to any association	83.5	80.4	84.6	77.5	97.6	94.0	96.4	93.7
Belong to other ethnic association	2.7	0.9	4.7	9.0	1.5	-	0.5	1.0
Total	100.0	100.0	100.0	100.0	100.0	100.0	100.0	100.0
Ethnicity of Close Friends								
All of own group	35.5	21.6	19.5	21.6	53.1	55.4	57.8	60.4
Some own group, some other	62.5	76.6	78.6	78.4	46.9	44.6	42.2	37.5
No close friends	2.0	1.8	1.9	-	-	-	-	2.1
Total	100.0	100.0	100.0	100.0	100.0	100.0	100.0	100.0

TABLE 3.6

Ethnic Attitudes towards Their Own Group and Other Ethnic Groups

	Chinese				Thai			
	Rural		Urban		Rural		Urban	
Variable	Female	Male	Female	Male	Female	Male	Female	Male
Ethnic Diversity Enriches a Nation's Culture	3.45	3.53	3.37	3.42	3.17	2.88	3.05	2.99
(Mean, Standard Deviation)	1.13	1.20	1.04	1.11	1.23	1.31	1.24	1.17
Intermarriage among Ethnic Groups should be Encouraged	3.13	3.37	3.25	3.45	2.84	2.81	2.90	2.88
(Mean, Standard Deviation)	1.06	0.99	0.95	0.99	1.15	1.09	1.11	1.11
It is Easier for (Own Group) to get Ahead these days	3.80	3.59	3.84	3.61	3.46	3.03	3.16	3.06
(Mean, Standard Deviation)	0.96	0.97	0.89	0.96	1.14	1.18	1.22	1.06
Ethnic Group is Strong if They are Many								
True	57.0	57.9	51.9	48.5	63.2	56.9	57.1	59.8
Depends	18.4	12.1	19.6	14.9	12.6	8.3	18.5	13.7
False	24.6	30.0	28.5	36.6	24.2	34.8	24.4	26.5
Total	100.0	100.0	100.0	100.0	100.0	100.0	100.0	100.0

TABLE 3.6 (cont'd)

Variable	Thai Muslim				Southern Thai Muslim			
	Rural		Urban		Rural		Urban	
	Female	Male	Female	Male	Female	Male	Female	Male
Ethnic Diversity Enriches a Nation's Culture	3.63	3.40	3.49	3.34	2.83	3.17	2.69	2.58
(Mean, Standard Deviation)	1.18	1.15	1.18	1.39	1.16	1.08	1.23	1.15
Intermarriage among Ethnic Groups should be Encouraged	2.89	3.17	2.92	3.11	2.28	2.25	2.21	2.16
(Mean, Standard Deviation)	1.28	1.09	1.23	1.24	1.07	0.87	1.12	1.16
It is Easier for (Own Group) to get Ahead these days	3.25	3.20	3.16	2.93	2.67	2.91	2.75	2.63
(Mean, Standard Deviation)	1.10	1.01	1.13	1.16	0.95	1.02	0.99	0.97
Ethnic Group is Strong if They are Many								
True	74.5	60.4	63.0	59.5	60.7	63.4	60.4	57.4
Depends	10.2	14.4	16.5	17.1	24.0	22.8	17.7	16.0
False	15.3	25.2	20.5	23.4	15.3	13.8	21.9	26.6
Total	100.0	100.0	100.0	100.0	100.0	100.0	100.0	100.0

TABLE 3.6 (cont'd)
Ethnic Attitudes towards Their Own Group and Other Ethnic Groups

	Chinese				Thai			
	Rural		Urban		Rural		Urban	
Variable	Female	Male	Female	Male	Female	Male	Female	Male
Socioeconomic Position of Ethnic Group is Better with								
Many children	11.1	5.7	7.3	12.7	8.7	7.3	6.8	3.0
Doesn't matter	9.2	13.2	12.0	15.7	7.5	5.5	10.5	16.8
Few children	79.7	81.1	80.7	71.6	83.8	87.2	82.7	80.2
Total	100.0	100.0	100.0	100.0	100.0	100.0	100.0	100.0
Mean Desirability as Friends Other Groups*	1.38	1.20	1.48	1.89	1.48	1.71	1.38	1.33
(Mean, Standard Deviation)	0.77	0.45	0.55	0.78	0.63	0.61	0.49	0.49
Mean Desirability Friends* Thai	2.44	2.42	2.35	2.47	2.85	2.79	2.62	2.69
(Mean, Standard Deviation)	0.52	0.53	0.52	0.58	0.37	0.41	0.50	0.47
Mean Desirability as Friends* Chinese	2.49	2.58	2.48	2.49	1.94	2.03	2.01	2.12
(Mean, Standard Deviation)	0.54	0.50	0.53	0.56	0.60	0.57	0.49	0.42
Mean Desirability as Friends* Thai Muslim	1.75	1.90	1.68	1.69	1.63	1.87	1.64	1.83
(Mean, Standard Deviation)	0.61	0.59	0.66	0.67	0.68	0.64	0.57	0.55

* 3-point scale.

TABLE 3.6 (cont'd)

Variable	Thai Muslim				Southern Thai Muslim			
	Rural		Urban		Rural		Urban	
	Female	Male	Female	Male	Female	Male	Female	Male
Socioeconomic Position of Ethnic Group is Better with								
Many children	16.5	14.3	11.7	20.9	24.4	17.8	25.4	25.5
Doesn't matter	14.8	16.1	13.6	13.6	15.2	13.9	8.8	10.6
Few children	68.7	69.6	74.7	65.5	60.4	68.3	65.8	63.9
Total	100.0	100.0	100.0	100.0	100.0	100.0	100.0	100.0
Mean Desirability as Friends Other Groups*	1.48	2.14	1.74	1.65	1.71	2.11	1.60	1.72
(Mean, Standard Deviation)	0.60	0.69	0.75	0.63	0.66	0.72	0.60	0.60
Mean Desirability Friends* Thai	2.27	2.42	2.39	2.46	1.92	2.17	2.08	2.17
(Mean, Standard Deviation)	0.59	0.53	0.58	0.54	0.53	0.68	0.54	0.52
Mean Desirability as Friends* Chinese	1.89	2.12	1.92	2.04	1.79	2.04	1.86	2.05
(Mean, Standard Deviation)	0.62	0.62	0.60	0.59	0.57	0.67	0.58	0.50
Mean Desirability as Friends* Thai Muslim	2.78	2.78	2.69	2.71	2.74	2.84	2.71	2.72
(Mean, Standard Deviation)	0.43	0.46	0.51	0.48	0.45	0.37	0.48	0.45

* 3-point scale.

TABLE 3.6 (cont'd)
Ethnic Attitudes towards Their Own Group and Other Ethnic Groups

Variable	Chinese				Thai			
	Rural		Urban		Rural		Urban	
	Female	Male	Female	Male	Female	Male	Female	Male
Mean Desirability as Friends*								
Southern Thai Muslim	1.63	1.72	1.52	1.92	1.59	1.58	1.58	1.25
(Mean, Standard Deviation)	0.55	0.46	0.55	0.79	0.64	0.61	0.54	0.45
Own Ethnic Group has								
Too many children	45.7	37.4	54.7	49.0	43.3	45.5	52.0	57.8
Right number	50.0	61.7	41.2	47.1	51.7	43.6	41.2	38.2
Too few children	4.3	0.9	4.1	3.9	5.0	10.9	6.8	4.0
Total	100.0	100.0	100.0	100.0	100.0	100.0	100.0	100.0
Ethnic Group with Largest Number of Children								
Chinese	51.3	37.9	54.3	62.7	42.5	52.7	53.4	59.0
Malay	-	-	-	-	-	-	0.3	-
Thai	22.5	26.2	23.6	17.6	36.6	31.8	29.8	29.0
Thai Muslim	21.2	28.2	16.6	16.7	17.8	13.7	12.7	11.0
Southern Thai Muslim	-	-	-	-	-	-	-	-
Burmese	-	-	-	-	-	0.9	-	-
Chinese and Thai about the same	0.7	-	0.3	1.0	0.3	-	1.6	-
About the same	4.3	7.7	5.2	2.0	1.6	0.9	2.2	-
Chinese and Islam about the same	-	-	-	-	0.6	-	-	1.0
Islam and Thai about the same	-	-	-	-	0.6	-	-	-
Total	100.0	100.0	100.0	100.0	100.0	100.0	100.0	100.0

* 3-point scale.

TABLE 3.6 (cont'd)

Variable	Thai Muslim				Southern Thai Muslim			
	Rural		Urban		Rural		Urban	
	Female	Male	Female	Male	Female	Male	Female	Male
Mean Desirability as Friends*								
Southern Thai Muslim	2.15	2.22	2.14	2.15	2.85	2.95	2.80	2.78
(Mean, Standard Deviation)	0.80	0.67	0.82	0.66	0.36	0.22	0.41	0.41
Own Ethnic Group has								
Too many children	46.4	33.9	45.4	32.4	55.8	70.3	57.1	61.1
Right number	48.2	57.2	49.5	64.0	42.6	27.7	41.9	35.8
Too few children	5.4	8.9	5.1	3.6	1.6	2.0	1.0	3.1
Total	100.0	100.0	100.0	100.0	100.0	100.0	100.0	100.0
Ethnic Group with Largest Number of Children								
Chinese	25.7	39.4	36.5	46.8	39.3	30.3	36.6	46.8
Malay	-	-	-	-	-	-	0.5	-
Thai	16.4	9.2	17.6	14.4	1.5	1.0	2.1	4.2
Thai Muslim	50.7	42.2	41.3	32.5	40.9	40.4	46.2	31.3
Southern Thai Muslim	1.4	-	-	-	16.3	28.3	13.6	16.7
Burmese	-	-	-	-	2.0	-	1.0	-
Chinese and Thai about the same	-	-	-	-	-	-	-	-
About the same	4.5	8.3	3.5	5.4	-	-	-	1.0
Chinese and Islam about the same	1.3	-	1.1	0.9	-	-	-	-
Islam and Thai about the same	-	0.9	-	-	-	-	-	-
Total	100.0	100.0	100.0	100.0	100.0	100.0	100.0	100.0

* 3-point scale.

The data also show that over half of the Southern Thai Muslims feel that the members of their own groups have too many children compared with less than half from the other ethnic groups who express a similar opinion. The urban members more readily admit that their own group has too many children compared with the rural counterparts.

Desirability as Friends

In rating the desirability of members of an ethnic group (on a 3-point rating scale) as friends, the data show that members of an ethnic group rate their fellow group members as more desirable friends than the members of the other groups. The score is highest among the Southern Thai Muslims, followed by the Thais, the Muslims and the Chinese respectively. The Chinese and the Southern Thai Muslims reciprocally find each other the least desirable. The Thais, apart from the preference for their own group, indicate that the Chinese are more favourable as friends than the Thai Muslims and the Southern Thai Muslims respectively. This preference probably reflects the greater cultural similarities of the Thais and the Thai Chinese.

When asked to identify an ethnic group with the largest number of children, half of the Chinese and about 40 per cent of the Thai Muslims in the South and in other parts of the country identify their own ethnic group as the most fertile. Only one-third of the Thai identify their own group as having the largest number of children. The Chinese are identified by no less than one-third of other ethnic groups as having the largest number of children, probably due to the image of the Chinese with their large family size in the past rather than actual knowledge of contemporary Chinese fertility behaviour. The Chinese at present rank second lowest after the Thais in terms of fertility. The differences in fertility and factors affecting it will be studied in the following chapters.

Contrasts of Demographic and Socio-Economic Characteristics of Ethnic Groups

Age

On an average husbands of all ethnic groups are older than their wives (Table 3.7). The average difference in the age of husbands and wives is greatest among the Southern Thai Muslims, about 6-7 years compared with an average of 5 years for the other ethnic groups. The average age of the Thai and the Thai Muslim husbands is about 36 years, compared with 37 years for the Southern Thai Muslims and 39 years for the Chinese.

The mean household size is smallest for the Thais, followed by the Southern Thai Muslims and the Thai Muslims. The Chinese have the largest household size.

Consistent with the findings on the household size, the data show that nuclear households are most prevalent among the Thais, but less prevalent among the Southern Thai Muslims, the Thai Muslims and the Chinese, respectively.

Educational Level

In terms of educational attainment, the husbands generally have more years of education than the wives. The urban couples are better educated than the rural ones (Table 3.8). In the urban areas, the Thai couples are best educated, followed by the Chinese, the Southern Thai Muslims and the Thai Muslims. In the rural areas, the Chinese couples are best educated, followed by the Southern Thai Muslims, the Thais and the Thai Muslims, respectively.

Sense of Efficacy and Control

When the respondents were asked about the relationship between luck and advancement in life, more rural people than urban people express the belief that "getting ahead in life is mostly a matter of luck". Strangely, more male than female respondents also believe likewise.

The Chinese as a group disagree more with the statement and obtain a higher score than the Thais and the Southern Thai Muslims, respectively. (The higher the score, the higher the sense of efficacy.) However, when the respondents were asked whether they felt they could control a lot of what happens in their lives, the Southern Thai Muslims score highest, followed by the Thais, the Thai Muslims and the Chinese. Male-female and urban-rural differences are minimal for all ethnic groups, except the Chinese. The discrepancies in answers for these two items probably indicate that they are not closely related from the point of view of the respondents.

TABLE 3.7

Residence, Age, Household Size and Composition by Ethnic Group

	Chinese				Thai			
	Rural		Urban		Rural		Urban	
Variable	Female	Male	Female	Male	Female	Male	Female	Male
Years Spent in Current Residence	18.70	23.92	15.43	18.83	17.79	15.95	14.94	17.13
(Mean, Standard Deviation)	12.75	13.86	11.87	13.93	12.43	12.00	11.73	12.53
Percentage of Life Spent in Cities	-	-	27.31	30.64	32.33	-	24.08	29.55
(Mean, Standard Deviation)	-	-	10.80	10.99	11.09	-	11.22	13.96
Age of Wife	33.59	33.70	33.41	31.78	31.76	32.56	31.43	31.86
(Mean, Standard Deviation)	6.69	6.85	6.15	6.45	7.21	7.05	7.00	7.15
Age of Husband	38.72	38.72	38.27	36.12	36.53	37.29	35.89	36.11
(Mean, Standard Deviation)	7.84	7.56	7.52	7.57	8.60	8.87	8.08	7.98
Household Size	6.89	6.75	6.95	6.51	5.58	5.56	5.59	5.72
(Mean, Standard Deviation)	4.39	3.03	3.59	3.84	2.56	2.36	2.42	2.15
Household Composition								
Nuclear	46.6	100.0	56.0	96.2	65.6	96.4	53.3	89.3
Extended with only one married couple	42.7	0.0	34.0	1.9	25.4	1.8	33.4	7.8
Extended with two or more married couples	10.7	0.0	10.0	1.9	9.0	1.8	13.3	2.9
Total	100.0	100.0	100.0	100.0	100.0	100.0	100.0	100.0

TABLE 3.7 (cont'd)

Variable	Thai Muslim				Southern Thai Muslim			
	Rural		Urban		Rural		Urban	
	Female	Male	Female	Male	Female	Male	Female	Male
Years Spent in Current Residence	17.72	20.61	17.41	20.45	21.95	24.45	17.70	19.88
(Mean, Standard Deviation)	12.55	13.31	12.31	16.32	12.50	14.75	12.23	15.77
Percentage of Life Spent in Cities	28.00	34.43	26.48	30.99	7.00	3.50	22.78	26.34
(Mean, Standard Deviation)	12.48	13.86	10.43	13.04	-	0.71	11.68	14.35
Age of Wife	31.15	31.64	31.38	31.34	30.53	30.28	30.31	30.60
(Mean, Standard Deviation)	7.36	7.35	7.16	7.07	8.47	7.97	7.57	8.15
Age of Husband	36.32	36.12	36.48	36.18	37.41	37.36	36.41	36.57
(Mean, Standard Deviation)	8.60	8.24	8.48	8.78	10.14	11.14	8.18	8.63
Household Size	6.55	6.85	6.98	6.79	5.84	5.59	6.64	6.72
(Mean, Standard Deviation)	3.43	4.07	3.37	3.25	2.75	2.87	4.76	4.42
Household Composition								
Nuclear	58.9	83.9	49.4	70.3	58.9	100.0	59.1	100.0
Extended with only one married couple	24.9	6.3	33.6	22.5	24.9	0.0	20.2	0.0
Extended with two or more married couples	16.2	9.8	17.0	7.2	16.2	0.0	20.7	0.0
Total	100.0	100.0	100.0	100.0	100.0	100.0	100.0	100.0

TABLE 3.8

Education and Sense of Efficacy and Control by Ethnic Group

	Chinese				Thai			
	Rural		Urban		Rural		Urban	
Variable	Female	Male	Female	Male	Female	Male	Female	Male
Education of Husband	7.55	7.51	8.55	8.63	6.60	7.30	8.92	9.49
(Mean years, Standard Deviation)	3.53	3.50	4.37	4.51	3.64	4.74	4.27	4.25
Education of Wife	6.22	6.32	6.93	6.67	5.51	5.76	7.12	6.81
(Mean years, Standard Deviation)	3.20	3.14	3.75	3.49	3.17	3.64	4.00	3.86
Getting Ahead in Life is Mostly a Matter of Luck*	2.69	3.06	2.93	3.03	2.53	3.16	2.77	3.23
(Mean, Standard Deviation)	1.26	1.36	1.20	1.30	1.23	1.37	1.31	1.30
You Feel you can Control A Lot of What Happens in your Life*	2.32	2.09	2.44	2.22	2.46	2.46	2.38	2.03
(Mean, Standard Deviation)	1.11	0.98	1.13	1.09	1.14	1.13	1.05	0.95

* 5-point scale.

TABLE 3.8 (cont'd)

Variable	Thai Muslim				Southern Thai Muslim			
	Rural		Urban		Rural		Urban	
	Female	Male	Female	Male	Female	Male	Female	Male
Education of Husband	6.10	6.59	7.86	8.07	6.65	7.00	7.39	7.14
(Mean years, Standard Deviation)	3.57	3.96	4.28	4.38	3.75	4.32	4.30	4.33
Education of Wife	5.27	5.44	6.66	6.51	6.57	6.90	7.06	7.43
(Mean years, Standard Deviation)	2.79	2.72	3.78	3.71	3.37	3.76	4.15	4.11
Getting Ahead in Life is Mostly a Matter of Luck*	2.55	2.88	2.70	3.06	2.60	2.30	2.65	2.73
(Mean, Standard Deviation)	1.31	1.33	1.33	1.45	1.11	0.90	1.18	1.22
You Feel you can Control A Lot of What Happens in your Life*	2.42	2.14	2.34	2.21	2.44	2.47	2.65	2.59
(Mean, Standard Deviation)	1.10	0.89	1.22	1.15	0.92	0.88	1.03	0.99

* 5-point scale.

Income and Wealth

Regarding the differences in income and wealth, the data show that the urban people generally have higher incomes than the rural people, and men earn more than women (Table 3.9). The Chinese on an average earn about Bht 5,000 compared with Bht 3,000, Bht 3,500, and Bht 2,500 earned by the Thais, the Thai Muslims and the Southern Thai Muslims, respectively. It is interesting to note that Thai wives earned more income than the wives of the Thai Muslims, the Chinese and the Southern Thai Muslims, respectively. The ratio of wives' income to husbands' income varied by ethnic group: two-fifths among the Thai, one-third among the Thai Muslim, one-fourth among the Southern Thai Muslim and one-sixth among the Chinese.

In the Thai social context, female employment in income earning activities is generally associated with the women's desire to earn additional income to support their families. This is enhanced by necessity or inadequacy of husband's earnings. The data consistently show that about one-third of the Chinese and the Southern Thai Muslim respondents, compared with more than 40 per cent of the Thais and the Thai Muslims, say that their family income is inadequate.

Home Ownership

With regard to home ownership, the data show that the percentage of home ownership of the urban people of all ethnic groups is lower than that of the rural people. No consistent male-female differences in home ownership are found. The percentage of home ownership is highest among the Southern Thai Muslims, followed by the Thai Muslims, the Thais, and the Chinese. More Chinese than Thais in the urban areas, however, own homes.

Possession of Consumer Durables

In terms of consumer durables, the Chinese score highest, followed by the Thais, then the Thai Muslims and the Southern Thai Muslims. To some extent, the possession of consumer durables reflects the different socio-economic position of the four ethnic groups.

Business Ownership and Type of Business

In terms of business ownership, other than farming and other wage earning activities, the Chinese have the highest score, followed by the Thai Muslims, the Thais and the Southern Thai Muslims. Over 60 per cent of the Chinese in both rural and urban areas are engaged in trade, wholesaling, retailing and hawking. Only one-fifth of the Thais and the two-fifths of the Thai Muslims are engaged in such businesses. The great majority of the Southern Thai Muslims do not own any business. They are probably farmers or rubber plantation workers. The data also show that the percentage of farm ownership is highest among the Southern Thai Muslims, the Thais and the Thai Muslims. However, it should be noted that the great majority of the rural respondents of all ethnic groups are not farmers. In the Thai rural areas, people can subsist by doing odd jobs as farming itself earns a very low income.

Support for/from Relatives

At least one-fifth of the respondents of all ethnic groups report that they provide some support for relatives. The highest percentage is reported by the Thai Muslims. This is followed by the Chinese, and the Southern Thai Muslims, and the Thais, respectively. The major recipients of the support in order of importance are the siblings of the wife or the husband, parents of the husband or the wife, and their own children.

The data also show that the highest proportion of the household heads who receive support from relatives is among the Southern Thai Muslims (22 per cent in the rural areas and 12.4 per cent in the urban areas). This is followed by the Thai Muslims, the Thais and the Chinese, respectively. The relatives who provide the support are consistently parents of the wife and the husband, and siblings of the wife or husband.

Husband's Occupation

About one-third of the Southern Thai Muslim husbands, compared with one-fourth of the Thai Muslims, one-fifth of the Thais and less than one-tenth of the Chinese are involved in farming, forestry and fishing (Table 3.10). Over 60 per cent of the Chinese husbands, compared with 28.7 per cent of the Thai Muslims, 24 per cent of the Southern Thai Muslims and 15 per cent of the Thais, are involved in sales.

TABLE 3.9

Income, Perceived Adequacy of Income, Assets, and Transfers of Economic Resources by Ethnic Groups

Variable	Chinese				Thai			
	Rural		Urban		Rural		Urban	
	Female	Male	Female	Male	Female	Male	Female	Male
Income of Husband	9.96	-	11.33	-	5.89	-	7.15	-
(Mean, Standard Deviation)	5.74	-	5.53	-	3.88	-	4.29	-
Income of Wife (Mean among Working Wives Only)	1.66	-	2.61	-	2.18	-	2.75	-
(Mean, Standard Deviation)	3.67	-	4.54	-	3.05	-	3.38	-
Perceived Adequacy of Family Income								
Inadequate	27.4	26.1	36.2	31.7	45.0	40.0	44.0	39.2
Just about adequate	64.5	69.2	57.5	59.6	50.3	59.1	50.8	58.8
More than adequate	8.1	4.7	6.3	8.7	4.7	0.9	5.2	2.0
Total	100.0	100.0	100.0	100.0	100.0	100.0	100.0	100.0
Home Ownership								
Owns	57.3	48.6	40.6	42.9	59.3	62.7	37.2	37.2
Rents	33.3	43.9	52.8	51.4	31.1	28.2	47.7	46.1
Other	9.4	7.5	6.6	5.7	9.6	9.1	15.1	16.7
Total	100.0	100.0	100.0	100.0	100.0	100.0	100.0	100.0

TABLE 3.9 (cont'd)

Variable	Thai Muslim				Southern Thai Muslim			
	Rural		Urban		Rural		Urban	
	Female	Male	Female	Male	Female	Male	Female	Male
Income of Husband	6.81	-	7.78	-	4.92	-	4.88	-
(Mean, Standard Deviation)	4.69	-	4.80	-	3.23	-	2.60	-
Income of Wife (Mean among Working Wives Only)	2.17	-	2.51	-	1.29	-	1.44	-
(Mean, Standard Deviation)	3.32	-	3.58	-	1.99	-	2.03	-
Perceived Adequacy of Family Income								
Inadequate	43.1	49.1	40.6	38.7	24.0	32.7	30.6	32.3
Just about adequate	52.2	47.3	54.7	57.7	73.0	61.4	63.7	64.6
More than adequate	4.7	3.6	4.7	3.6	3.0	5.9	5.7	3.1
Total	100.0	100.0	100.0	100.0	100.0	100.0	100.0	100.0
Home Ownership								
Owns	73.7	71.4	50.6	53.2	75.6	69.3	59.1	64.6
Rents	12.8	12.5	31.8	31.5	18.8	20.8	31.6	25.0
Other	13.5	16.1	17.6	15.3	5.6	9.9	9.3	10.4
Total	100.0	100.0	100.0	100.0	100.0	100.0	100.0	100.0

TABLE 3.9 (cont'd)
Income, Perceived Adequacy of Income, Assets, and Transfers of Economic Resources by Ethnic Groups

Variable	Chinese				Thai			
	Rural		Urban		Rural		Urban	
	Female	Male	Female	Male	Female	Male	Female	Male
Business Ownership								
Owns	76.5	85.0	79.2	86.7	38.5	41.8	37.2	49.0
Does not own	23.5	15.0	20.8	13.3	61.5	58.2	62.8	51.0
Total	100.0	100.0	100.0	100.0	100.0	100.0	100.0	100.0
Type of Business (Percentage Based on Owners Only)								
Does not own business	23.5	15.0	20.9	13.3	61.2	57.8	62.5	51.0
Agriculture agro-business	3.3	0.9	0.9	-	0.6	1.8	0.9	1.0
Trade, wholesale	3.6	4.7	1.4	1.0	0.9	0.9	1.9	2.0
Trade, retail hawking	60.9	65.4	67.4	73.3	23.0	29.4	17.0	31.2
Handicrafts	2.3	2.8	0.6	-	3.7	0.9	6.8	-
Manufacturing	2.9	7.5	2.8	3.8	3.7	4.6	3.4	5.9
Services	2.0	3.7	3.2	5.7	5.0	3.7	6.2	6.9
Transport	0.3	-	0.3	-	0.7	-	0.6	1.0
Other	1.2	-	2.5	2.9	1.2	0.9	0.7	1.0
Total	100.0	100.0	100.0	100.0	100.0	100.0	100.0	100.0
Farm Ownership								
Owner	1.7	-	-	-	5.7	7.3	0.9	1.0
Tenant	0.3	-	0.3	1.0	6.9	5.5	0.3	-
Hired labourer	-	-	-	-	2.2	1.8	-	-
Nonfarm	97.7	100.0	99.4	99.0	84.6	84.5	98.8	99.0
Other	0.3	-	0.3	-	0.6	0.9	-	-
Total	100.0	100.0	100.0	100.0	100.0	100.0	100.0	100.0
Size of Farm (Mean Hectares among Owners only)	0.10	-	-	-	0.72	0.51	0.07	0.08
(Mean, Standard Deviation)	0.88	-	-	-	4.94	2.04	0.68	0.79

TABLE 3.9 (cont'd)

Variable	Thai Muslim				Southern Thai Muslim			
	Rural		Urban		Rural		Urban	
	Female	Male	Female	Male	Female	Male	Female	Male
Business Ownership								
Owns	49.2	62.5	51.3	47.7	12.2	9.0	12.4	12.5
Does not own	50.8	37.5	48.7	52.3	87.8	91.0	87.6	87.5
Total	100.0	100.0	100.0	100.0	100.0	100.0	100.0	100.0
Type of Business (Percentage Based on Owners Only)								
Does not own business	50.8	37.8	48.4	52.3	87.3	90.0	87.0	86.5
Agriculture agro-business	2.0	0.9	1.3	0.9	-	1.0	0.5	-
Trade, wholesale	1.3	-	2.5	-	1.0	1.0	2.1	4.1
Trade, retail hawking	41.8	53.2	42.5	41.4	3.6	6.0	8.8	7.3
Handicrafts	0.3	0.9	0.9	0.9	5.6	1.0	1.6	2.1
Manufacturing	2.5	3.6	2.2	1.8	-	-	-	-
Services	0.3	0.9	0.9	0.9	1.0	-	-	-
Transport	0.3	-	-	-	1.0	-	-	-
Other	0.7	2.7	1.3	1.8	0.5	1.0	-	-
Total	100.0	100.0	100.0	100.0	100.0	100.0	100.0	100.0
Farm Ownership								
Owner	6.1	4.6	0.3	-	11.6	13.8	2.7	2.2
Tenant	4.8	3.7	0.3	-	3.3	-	-	-
Hired labourer	1.4	1.8	-	-	0.6	1.1	-	-
Nonfarm	87.4	88.1	99.4	-	84.5	85.1	97.3	97.8
Other	0.3	1.8	-	-	-	-	-	-
Total	100.0	100.0	100.0	100.0	100.0	100.0	100.0	100.0
Size of Farm (Mean Hectares among Owners only)	0.29	0.32	0.06	-	1.11	2.05	0.12	0.17
(Mean, Standard Deviation)	1.43	1.51	1.12	-	9.12	12.63	0.88	1.21

TABLE 3.9 (cont'd)
Income, Perceived Adequacy of Income, Assets, and
Transfers of Economic Resources by Ethnic Groups

	Chinese				Thai			
	Rural		Urban		Rural		Urban	
Variable	Female	Male	Female	Male	Female	Male	Female	Male
Support Provided for Relatives								
No	77.2	72.9	76.1	80.0	80.7	79.1	80.7	77.5
Yes	22.8	27.1	23.9	20.0	19.3	20.9	19.3	22.5
Total	100.0	100.0	100.0	100.0	100.0	100.0	100.0	100.0
Number of Consumer Durables Owned	6.80	7.08	7.54	7.29	4.56	4.86	5.77	5.87
(Mean, Standard Deviation)	3.77	1.83	2.57	1.78	2.68	2.10	4.18	1.94
Relatives who Receive Support								
Parents of wife	15.7	-	25.0	23.9	25.4	8.7	25.4	4.3
Parents of husband	21.5	24.2	13.2	19.0	12.7	21.7	19.0	21.8
Children	10.0	10.3	9.2	9.5	7.9	13.0	1.6	-
Siblings of wife or husband	51.4	65.5	51.3	47.6	54.0	56.6	54.0	73.9
Other	1.4	-	1.3	-	-	-	-	-
Total	100.0	100.0	100.0	100.0	100.0	100.0	100.0	100.0
Support Received from Relatives								
No	87.3	87.9	88.7	88.6	84.1	80.0	82.9	76.5
Yes	12.7	12.1	11.3	11.4	15.9	20.0	17.1	23.5
Total	100.0	100.0	100.0	100.0	100.0	100.0	100.0	100.0

TABLE 3.9 (cont'd)

Variable	Thai Muslim				Southern Thai Muslim			
	Rural		Urban		Rural		Urban	
	Female	Male	Female	Male	Female	Male	Female	Male
Support Provided for Relatives								
No	74.7	79.5	73.3	69.4	76.6	81.2	80.3	76.0
Yes	25.3	20.5	26.7	30.6	23.4	18.8	19.7	24.0
Total	100.0	100.0	100.0	100.0	100.0	100.0	100.0	100.0
Number of Consumer Durables Owned	4.37	4.91	5.78	5.71	4.37	4.63	4.68	5.03
(Mean, Standard Deviation)	2.40	2.42	2.32	2.32	2.30	2.37	2.22	2.21
Relatives who Receive Support								
Parents of wife	25.0	13.0	29.4	17.6	19.6	5.0	31.6	30.4
Parents of husband	10.5	26.1	15.3	38.3	6.5	20.0	10.5	17.4
Children	7.9	13.0	5.9	-	-	-	13.2	8.7
Siblings of wife or husband	53.9	47.9	49.4	44.1	73.9	75.0	44.7	43.5
Other	2.7	-	-	-	-	-	-	-
Total	100.0	100.0	100.0	100.0	100.0	100.0	100.0	100.0
Support Received from Relatives								
No	79.5	83.9	85.5	81.1	77.7	84.2	87.6	86.5
Yes	20.5	16.1	14.5	18.9	22.3	15.8	12.4	13.5
Total	100.0	100.0	100.0	100.0	100.0	100.0	100.0	100.0

TABLE 3.9 (cont'd)
Income, Perceived Adequacy of Income, Assets, and
Transfers of Economic Resources by Ethnic Groups

Variable	Chinese				Thai			
	Rural		Urban		Rural		Urban	
	Female	Male	Female	Male	Female	Male	Female	Male
Relatives who Provide Support								
Parents of wife	23.1	-	25.0	8.3	28.2	9.1	33.9	4.2
Parents of husband	10.3	15.4	8.3	16.7	13.2	27.3	1.8	8.3
Children	5.1	-	5.6	-	5.7	-	7.1	8.3
Sibling of wife or husband	61.5	76.9	61.1	75.0	49.1	63.6	57.2	79.2
Other	-	7.7	-	-	3.8	-	-	-
Total	100.0	100.0	100.0	100.0	100.0	100.0	100.0	100.0

TABLE 3.9 (cont'd)

Variable	Thai Muslim				Southern Thai Muslim			
	Rural		Urban		Rural		Urban	
	Female	Male	Female	Male	Female	Male	Female	Male
Relatives who Provide Support								
Parents of wife	24.3	5.6	28.3	4.8	20.0	29.4	45.8	38.5
Parents of husband	4.8	22.2	13.0	23.8	13.3	23.5	4.2	7.7
Children	4.8	11.1	2.2	-	4.4	5.9	-	-
Sibling of wife or husband	62.9	50.0	56.5	71.4	57.8	29.4	50.0	53.8
Other	3.2	11.1	-	-	4.5	11.8	-	-
Total	100.0	100.0	100.0	100.0	100.0	100.0	100.0	100.0

TABLE 3.10

Employment Characteristics by Ethnic Group

Variable	Chinese				Thai			
	Rural		Urban		Rural		Urban	
	Female	Male	Female	Male	Female	Male	Female	Male
Husband's Occupation								
Professional, technical	2.0	0.9	1.3	1.0	4.4	8.2	7.4	9.8
Administrative, managerial	1.3	0.9	2.8	1.0	11.5	11.8	14.6	14.7
Clerical	3.0	1.9	5.0	3.8	4.7	4.5	6.2	6.9
Sales	60.6	77.6	67.6	74.2	14.6	18.2	18.6	24.5
Service	14.1	4.7	8.2	6.6	28.0	21.8	30.7	25.5
Production, transport, labourers	7.1	8.4	11.3	12.4	14.0	13.7	14.5	13.7
Farm, forestry, fishing	8.9	3.7	1.3	-	18.7	18.2	5.8	2.9
Unemployed	0.7	-	1.6	1.0	1.9	2.7	-	-
Occupation not elsewhere classified	2.3	1.9	0.9	-	2.2	0.9	2.2	2.0
Total	100.0	100.0	100.0	100.0	100.0	100.0	100.0	100.0

TABLE 3.10 (cont'd)

Variable	Thai Muslim				Southern Thai Muslim			
	Rural		Urban		Rural		Urban	
	Female	Male	Female	Male	Female	Male	Female	Male
Husband's Occupation								
Professional, technical	3.4	2.7	8.2	9.0	4.1	6.8	6.3	5.2
Administrative, managerial	3.4	4.5	5.7	7.2	5.1	5.0	6.3	8.3
Clerical	1.7	4.5	6.9	6.3	2.5	1.0	2.5	3.1
Sales	28.7	39.3	41.5	46.8	24.4	23.8	21.4	19.8
Service	22.0	16.1	21.4	18.0	17.8	16.8	27.6	33.3
Production, transport, labourers	10.4	9.8	8.8	7.3	10.2	10.9	20.3	12.6
Farm, forestry, fishing	25.6	18.8	3.5	3.6	32.5	29.7	13.0	14.6
Unemployed	2.4	2.6	2.7	0.9	1.0	1.0	1.6	1.0
Occupation not elsewhere classified	2.4	1.7	1.3	0.9	2.4	5.0	1.0	2.1
Total	100.0	100.0	100.0	100.0	100.0	100.0	100.0	100.0

TABLE 3.10 (cont'd)
Employment Characteristics by Ethnic Group

Variable	Chinese				Thai			
	Rural		Urban		Rural		Urban	
	Female	Male	Female	Male	Female	Male	Female	Male
Wife's Employment								
Currently employed	78.8	77.5	79.2	77.1	66.8	73.6	65.0	65.6
Not currently employed but has worked since marriage	2.9	4.7	5.3	7.6	8.7	7.3	7.7	6.9
Not employed since marriage	18.3	17.8	15.5	15.3	24.5	19.1	27.3	27.5
Total	100.0	100.0	100.0	100.0	100.0	100.0	100.0	100.0
Length of Time since Marriage Wife has been Employed (Mean years for all Wives)	8.48	-	7.98	-	6.32	-	5.81	-
(Mean, Standard Deviation)	7.74	-	7.23	-	7.20	-	6.66	-

TABLE 3.10 (cont'd)

Variable	Thai Muslim				Southern Thai Muslim			
	Rural		Urban		Rural		Urban	
	Female	Male	Female	Male	Female	Male	Female	Male
Wife's Employment								
Currently employed	64.6	65.2	68.2	68.5	53.3	60.4	47.2	43.8
Not currently employed but has worked since marriage	9.1	7.1	9.2	5.4	4.6	4.0	4.1	4.2
Not employed since marriage	26.3	27.7	22.6	26.1	42.1	35.6	48.7	52.0
Total	100.0	100.0	100.0	100.0	100.0	100.0	100.0	100.0
Length of Time since Marriage Wife has been Employed (Mean years for all Wives)	6.31	-	6.43	-	6.82	-	5.44	-
(Mean, Standard Deviation)	1.59	-	7.44	-	9.16	-	8.86	-

TABLE 3.10 (cont'd)
Employment Characteristics by Ethnic Group

Variable	Chinese				Thai			
	Rural		Urban		Rural		Urban	
	Female	Male	Female	Male	Female	Male	Female	Male
Wife's Occupation (Percentage Based on Wives Who have Worked since Marriage)								
Professional, technical	2.3	2.8	1.3	1.9	3.1	4.5	7.7	4.9
Administrative, managerial	-	-	0.9	1.9	2.2	3.6	5.0	4.9
Clerical	1.0	1.9	2.2	2.9	1.2	2.7	2.8	3.9
Sales	62.9	65.4	65.3	68.3	28.7	36.4	28.2	36.3
Service	0.6	-	4.4	2.9	12.8	11.9	15.8	9.7
Production, transport, Labourers	7.5	8.4	8.6	5.8	8.4	9.1	8.4	10.8
Farm, forestry, fishing	6.2	1.9	0.3	-	15.0	12.7	1.5	1.0
Unemployed	19.2	19.6	17.0	16.3	28.3	19.1	29.4	27.5
Occupation not elsewhere classified	0.3	-	-	-	0.3	-	1.2	1.0
Total	100.0	100.0	100.0	100.0	100.0	100.0	100.0	100.0

TABLE 3.10 (cont'd)

Variable	Thai Muslim				Southern Thai Muslim			
	Rural		Urban		Rural		Urban	
	Female	Male	Female	Male	Female	Male	Female	Male
Wife's Occupation (Percentage Based on Wives Who have Worked since Marriage)								
Professional, technical	2.4	1.8	6.0	4.5	4.1	5.9	3.1	1.0
Administrative, managerial	0.7	1.8	3.5	4.5	1.5	1.0	1.5	2.1
Clerical	0.7	0.9	1.9	1.8	0.5	1.0	-	-
Sales	40.4	42.0	50.9	45.9	28.3	26.7	33.2	32.3
Service	7.6	6.1	4.7	4.6	1.5	2.0	5.2	5.2
Production, transport, Labourers	5.1	4.5	5.3	8.1	7.7	7.9	5.2	4.2
Farm, forestry, fishing	12.5	11.6	2.2	1.8	14.9	20.8	2.1	2.1
Unemployed	30.6	31.3	25.5	28.8	41.5	34.7	49.2	53.1
Occupation not elsewhere classified	-	-	-	-	-	-	0.5	-
Total	100.0	100.0	100.0	100.0	100.0	100.0	100.0	100.0

TABLE 3.10 (cont'd)
Employment Characteristics by Ethnic Group

	Chinese				Thai			
	Rural		Urban		Rural		Urban	
Variable	Female	Male	Female	Male	Female	Male	Female	Male
Location of Wife's Work								
At home	66.4	67.4	67.8	67.3	29.5	30.0	29.7	28.4
Nearby	9.8	12.1	11.0	10.6	28.5	33.6	26.6	30.4
Far from home	4.6	0.9	3.8	4.8	13.7	17.3	14.6	13.7
Never worked	19.2	19.6	17.4	17.3	28.3	19.1	29.1	27.5
Total	100.0	100.0	100.0	100.0	100.0	100.0	100.0	100.0
Wife's Employer								
Self employed	48.2	47.7	51.1	49.0	29.5	30.9	29.8	26.4
Family member	26.1	27.1	21.5	26.9	20.5	19.1	13.9	20.6
Someone else	6.5	5.6	10.4	7.7	21.7	30.9	26.9	25.5
Never worked	19.2	19.6	17.0	16.4	28.3	19.1	29.4	27.5
Total	100.0	100.0	100.0	100.0	100.0	100.0	100.0	100.0

TABLE 3.10 (cont'd)

Variable	Thai Muslim				Southern Thai Muslim			
	Rural		Urban		Rural		Urban	
	Female	Male	Female	Male	Female	Male	Female	Male
Location of Wife's Work								
At home	24.6	25.0	24.0	27.1	29.9	30.6	26.9	22.9
Nearby	34.0	33.0	31.5	28.8	18.3	19.8	13.5	14.6
Far from home	10.4	10.7	18.9	16.2	10.7	14.9	10.9	9.4
Never worked	31.0	31.3	25.6	27.9	41.1	34.7	48.7	53.1
Total	100.0	100.0	100.0	100.0	100.0	100.0	100.0	100.0
Wife's Employer								
Self employed	36.4	32.1	35.8	39.6	38.8	44.0	31.1	29.2
Family member	20.2	25.0	19.8	18.0	11.2	12.0	14.5	12.5
Someone else	12.8	11.6	18.9	13.6	8.7	8.0	5.2	5.2
Never worked	30.6	31.3	25.5	28.8	41.3	36.0	49.2	53.1
Total	100.0	100.0	100.0	100.0	100.0	100.0	100.0	100.0

Wife's Employment

There are also significant differences in wife's employment among the ethnic groups. The percentage of working wives is highest among the Chinese (over 75 per cent), followed by the Thais, the Thai Muslims and the Southern Thai Muslims, respectively. Chinese wives also record the longest length of working time, followed by the Southern Thai Muslims, the Thais and the Thai Muslims respectively. Among the working wives, over 60 per cent of the Chinese are in sales compared with less than one-third of the Thai and Southern Thai Muslim wives and two-fifths of the Thai Muslims wives.

Over two-thirds of the Chinese wives, compared with one-third of the wives of the other three ethnic groups, work at home as they are self- or family-employed. It is interesting to note that the percentage of wives working far from home is highest among the Thais and lowest among the Chinese. Only one-tenth of the Thai Muslim wives in all parts of the country work far from home.

In brief, there are significant differences among the Chinese, the Thais, the Thai Muslims and the Southern Thai Muslims in ethnicity-related variables and in demographic and socio-economic characteristics. The differences reflect largely social and cultural differences of the respective ethnic groups.

IV

ETHNIC DIFFERENCES IN FERTILITY, FAMILY PLANNING AND RELATED VARIABLES

The comparative description of ethnic, demographic and socio-economic characteristics of the four major ethnic groups presented in the previous chapter provides some background to the understanding of analysis of ethnic fertility differentials and factors affecting them. The present chapter will present the pattern of ethnic fertility differentials and the differences in factors affecting them. Among the factors are fertility preferences, preference for children of a given sex, value of children, family planning knowledge, attitudes and practice, variables related to marriage and divorce and the type and pattern of spouse interactions.

Differences in Fertility

Pregnancies, Live Births and Living Children

The statistics clearly show that the Thai Muslims in various parts of the country and the Southern Thai Muslims have higher fertility than the Thais and the Chinese. The average number of live births in the rural areas is 3.03 for the Thais, 3.29 for the Chinese, 3.49 for the Southern Thai Muslims and 3.80 for the Thai Muslims (Table 4.1). The urban members of each ethnic group average fewer pregnancies and live births than their rural counterparts. The patterns of differences in the number of pregnancies, living children and children who died remain consistently the same among the ethnic groups.

Miscarriages, Still Births and Abortions

Regarding miscarriages and still births, the Thais and the Thai Muslims have a higher average than the Chinese and the Southern Thai Muslims, respectively. The Thais and the Chinese also report a higher rate of abortions than the Thai Muslims in the South and in other parts of the country.

Living Sons and Daughters, and Children Living Away

With a greater number of live births, the Thai Muslims and the Southern Thai Muslims also have a greater number of living sons than the Chinese and the Thais respectively. The Thais average the smallest number of living daughters; the Thai Muslims average the greatest number. The Chinese have a slightly greater number of daughters than the Southern Thai Muslims. The number of children living in the Chinese households is greater than those in the Southern Thai Muslim and the Thai households, even though the Chinese have a lower number of live births and living children than the Southern Thai Muslims. Also, the Chinese parents are inclined towards having their daughters stay at home. For all ethnic groups, the number of children living away is greater among the rural than the urban households.

Children from Previous Sexual Union and Adopted Children

The percentage of households with children from a previous sexual union is highest among the Southern Thai Muslims, followed by the Thais, the Thai Muslims and lowest among the Chinese. Similarly too, the Chinese average a lower percentage of households with adopted children than the Thai Muslims, the Thais and the Southern Thai Muslims.

Age of Eldest and Youngest Children

The mean age of the eldest children ranges from 12.4 years among the rural Chinese to 18.4 years among the rural Thai Muslims. The range of mean age of the youngest children is from 5.87 among the Thai Muslims to 12.45 among the Southern Thai Muslims. To some extent, the higher the age of the eldest child the earlier the family formation of the ethnic group. However, one must also look into other factors such as the first birth interval and current age of the couples.

TABLE 4.1
Fertility and Fertility Preferences by Ethnic Group

Variable	Chinese				Thai			
	Rural		Urban		Rural		Urban	
	Female	Male	Female	Male	Female	Male	Female	Male
Total Pregnancies	3.31	-	3.07	-	3.10	-	2.78	-
(Mean, Standard Deviation)	1.98	-	1.93	-	2.35	-	1.75	-
Children Ever Born	3.29	3.22	3.05	2.96	3.03	3.14	2.67	2.73
(Mean, Standard Deviation)	1.75	1.60	1.69	1.82	1.95	1.98	1.53	1.51
Living Children	3.25	3.12	2.99	2.92	2.87	3.01	2.60	2.66
(Mean, Standard Deviation)	2.28	1.51	1.66	1.81	1.81	1.82	1.47	1.46
Children Who Died	0.17	-	0.07	-	0.20	-	0.09	0.04
(Mean, Standard Deviation)	0.51	-	0.28	-	0.64	-	0.32	0.24
Miscarriages	0.14	-	0.18	-	0.24	-	0.17	-
(Mean, Standard Deviation)	0.46	-	0.55	-	0.73	-	0.52	-
Still Births	0.01	-	0.01	-	0.02	-	0.01	-
(Mean, Standard Deviation)	0.06	-	0.08	-	0.19	-	0.10	-
Abortions	0.02	-	0.03	-	0.02	-	0.02	-
(Mean, Standard Deviation)	0.15	-	0.27	-	0.21	-	0.21	-
Living Sons	1.83	1.74	1.62	1.68	1.66	1.65	1.56	1.67
(Mean, Standard Deviation)	1.13	1.14	1.30	1.37	1.42	1.44	1.19	1.17

TABLE 4.1 (cont'd)

Variable	Thai Muslim				Southern Thai Muslim			
	Rural		Urban		Rural		Urban	
	Female	Male	Female	Male	Female	Male	Female	Male
Total Pregnancies	3.98	-	3.34	-	3.53	-	3.78	-
(Mean, Standard Deviation)	2.88	-	2.61	-	2.45	-	2.56	-
Children Ever Born	3.80	3.99	3.25	3.24	3.49	3.61	3.66	3.75
(Mean, Standard Deviation)	2.51	2.72	2.24	2.18	2.19	2.40	2.42	2.47
Living Children	3.69	3.65	3.03	3.07	3.23	3.28	3.44	3.61
(Mean, Standard Deviation)	2.30	2.34	1.95	1.91	1.97	2.04	2.15	2.31
Children Who Died	0.33	0.11	0.21	0.04	0.26	-	0.23	0.01
(Mean, Standard Deviation)	0.81	0.49	0.62	0.28	0.65	-	0.60	0.10
Miscarriages	0.22	-	0.29	-	0.04	-	0.07	-
(Mean, Standard Deviation)	0.60	-	0.73	-	0.20	-	0.29	-
Still Births	0.02	-	-	-	0.05	-	0.03	-
(Mean, Standard Deviation)	0.16	-	0.06	-	0.32	-	0.16	-
Abortions	-	-	0.01	-	0.01	-	-	-
(Mean, Standard Deviation)	-	-	0.11	-	0.07	-	-	-
Living Sons	2.17	2.05	1.67	1.64	1.87	1.94	1.88	2.04
(Mean, Standard Deviation)	1.67	1.58	1.28	1.27	1.43	1.43	1.29	1.37

TABLE 4.1 (cont'd)
Fertility and Fertility Preferences by Ethnic Group

Variable	Chinese				Thai			
	Rural		Urban		Rural		Urban	
	Female	Male	Female	Male	Female	Male	Female	Male
Living Daughters	1.42	1.38	1.37	1.24	1.21	2.36	1.04	0.99
(Mean, Standard Deviation)	1.38	1.21	1.17	1.14	1.25	1.23	1.01	0.97
Children Living in Household	2.65	-	2.65	-	2.38	-	2.14	-
(Mean, Standard Deviation)	1.69	-	1.71	-	0.73	-	1.42	-
Children Living Away	0.69	-	0.34	-	0.49	-	0.46	-
(Mean, Standard Deviation)	0.72	-	0.52	-	0.81	-	0.58	-
Percentage with Children from Previous Sexual Union	-	1.8	0.3	3.0	4.6	9.1	3.1	5.0
Percentage with Adopted Children	5.5	8.4	4.4	2.9	7.4	10.9	6.2	6.9
Age of Eldest	13.98	-	12.42	-	14.88	-	12.15	-
(Mean, Standard Deviation)	18.39	-	15.93	-	20.60	-	16.05	-
Age of Youngest	7.24	-	6.83	-	8.91	-	7.23	-
(Mean, Standard Deviation)	13.22	-	11.35	-	16.71	-	11.85	-
Length of 1st Interval								
Mean	22.4	-	19.6	-	20.0	-	19.9	-
Standard Deviation	39.6	-	16.5	-	13.8	-	17.2	-
Total	280	-	293	-	287	-	284	-

TABLE 4.1 (cont'd)

Variable	Thai Muslim				Southern Thai Muslim			
	Rural		Urban		Rural		Urban	
	Female	Male	Female	Male	Female	Male	Female	Male
Living Daughters	1.52	1.60	1.36	1.43	1.36	1.34	1.56	1.57
(Mean, Standard Deviation)	1.47	1.58	1.37	1.75	1.37	1.29	1.44	1.43
Children Living in Househol	2.89	-	2.54	-	2.56	-	2.80	-
(Mean, Standard Deviation)	2.16	-	1.92	-	1.94	-	2.12	-
Children Living Away	0.08	0.09	0.49	0.02	0.67	-	0.64	0.04
(Mean, Standard Deviation)	0.94	0.49	0.72	0.19	0.61	-	0.82	0.41
Percentage with Children from Previous Sexual Union	4.4	9.8	3.1	7.2	6.1	4.0	6.2	8.3
Percentage with Adopted Children	7.1	8.9	7.6	11.7	11.7	14.9	7.8	11.5
Age of Eldest	18.40	-	13.90	-	17.64	-	12.73	-
(Mean, Standard Deviation)	25.31	-	19.76	-	21.74	-	13.76	-
Age of Youngest	5.87	-	8.44	-	12.45	-	7.11	-
(Mean, Standard Deviation)	11.56	-	15.77	-	24.90	-	16.67	-
Length of 1st Interval								
Mean	21.4	-	21.3	-	31.0	-	27.8	-
Standard Deviation	19.7	-	18.1	-	36.1	-	30.8	-
Total	251	-	285	-	165	-	167	-

TABLE 4.1 (cont'd)
Fertility and Fertility Preferences by Ethnic Group

	Chinese				Thai			
	Rural		Urban		Rural		Urban	
Variable	Female	Male	Female	Male	Female	Male	Female	Male
Length of 2nd Interval								
Mean	26.8	-	26.0	-	27.9	-	30.8	-
Standard Deviation	20.9	-	16.6	-	15.9	-	17.4	-
Total	236	-	237	-	223	-	214	-
Percentage Currently Pregnant	8.5	16.8	11.3	12.5	8.7	3.7	5.0	4.9
Ideal Family Size	3.35	3.50	3.21	3.46	2.90	3.08	2.70	2.81
(Mean, Standard Deviation)	1.08	1.25	1.19	1.41	1.08	1.36	1.05	1.09
Ideal Number of Sons	1.74	1.90	1.62	1.87	1.38	1.61	1.36	1.66
(Mean, Standard Deviation)	0.85	0.97	1.02	1.09	0.80	1.21	0.89	1.18
Ideal Number of Daughters	1.39	1.36	1.37	1.32	1.32	1.44	1.23	1.23
(Mean, Standard Deviation)	0.74	0.83	0.92	0.88	0.84	1.13	0.84	1.04
Desired Family Size	3.42	3.70	3.28	3.68	3.13	3.35	2.88	3.16
(Mean, Standard Deviation)	1.46	1.44	1.41	1.63	1.44	1.59	1.28	1.33
Additional Number of Children Desired	0.65	0.78	0.59	1.08	0.59	0.78	0.62	0.71
(Mean, Standard Deviation)	1.12	1.14	0.98	1.48	0.85	1.22	0.86	0.91

TABLE 4.1 (cont'd)

Variable	Thai Muslim				Southern Thai Muslim			
	Rural		Urban		Rural		Urban	
	Female	Male	Female	Male	Female	Male	Female	Male
Length of 2nd Interval								
Mean	27.8	-	24.9	-	35.1	-	30.6	-
Standard Deviation	16.2	-	17.6	-	25.0	-	18.5	-
Total	222	-	223	-	124	-	135	-
Percentage Currently Pregnant	8.8	5.5	6.7	6.5	5.1	4.0	9.0	8.4
Ideal Family Size	3.35	3.66	3.17	3.70	3.75	3.60	3.44	3.56
(Mean, Standard Deviation)	1.41	1.86	1.29	1.61	1.44	1.38	1.27	1.49
Ideal Number of Sons	1.74	2.25	1.67	2.03	1.83	2.00	1.74	2.06
(Mean, Standard Deviation)	1.02	1.62	1.10	1.20	0.95	1.17	0.90	1.28
Ideal Number of Daughters	1.53	1.57	1.43	1.48	1.82	1.68	1.59	1.54
(Mean, Standard Deviation)	0.87	1.24	1.00	1.08	1.02	1.17	0.89	1.14
Desired Family Size	3.80	4.15	3.35	3.70	3.66	3.65	3.47	3.54
(Mean, Standard Deviation)	1.82	2.12	1.56	1.66	1.96	2.19	2.10	2.30
Additional Number of Children Desired	0.89	1.28	0.98	1.26	1.35	1.54	0.98	1.05
(Mean, Standard Deviation)	1.26	1.92	1.34	1.67	1.54	1.73	1.33	1.30

TABLE 4.1 (cont'd)
Fertility and Fertility Preferences by Ethnic Group

	Chinese				Thai			
	Rural		Urban		Rural		Urban	
Variable	Female	Male	Female	Male	Female	Male	Female	Male
Additional Children								
Desired by Spouse	0.60	0.63	0.56	0.77	0.65	0.74	0.58	0.62
(Mean, Standard Deviation)	1.16	1.14	0.95	1.15	1.03	1.32	1.02	0.93
Number of Sons Desired								
Given Exactly 3 Children	1.80	1.88	1.82	1.90	1.59	1.78	1.66	1.85
(Mean, Standard Deviation)	0.49	0.36	0.51	0.54	0.52	0.60	0.55	0.50

TABLE 4.1 (cont'd)

Variable	Thai Muslim				Southern Thai Muslim			
	Rural		Urban		Rural		Urban	
	Female	Male	Female	Male	Female	Male	Female	Male
Additional Children Desired by Spouse (Mean, Standard Deviation)	0.77 1.30	0.70 1.15	0.73 1.22	1.04 1.64	0.75 1.19	0.74 1.16	0.51 1.00	0.58 1.21
Number of Sons Desired Given Exactly 3 Children (Mean, Standard Deviation)	1.67 0.60	1.76 0.51	1.68 0.60	1.88 0.49	1.60 0.52	1.76 0.50	1.60 0.53	1.74 0.47

First and Second Birth Intervals

The data show that the first birth interval is longest among the Southern Thai Muslims, followed by the Thai Muslims, the Thais and the Chinese. The fact that the Southern Thai Muslims and the Thai Muslims end up by having a greater family size implies that they do not practice contraception except perhaps to delay pregnancy immediately after marriage as evidenced by the longer first birth intervals. The longer interval between marriage and first birth could also be due to the fact that the Muslims marry very young before their prime fecundity. Otherwise, their family size would be much greater or closer to that of natural fertility. The statistics also show that the percentage of women currently pregnant is highest among the Thai Muslims. This is followed by the Thais, the Chinese and the Southern Thai Muslims respectively.

Differences in Fertility Preferences, Sex Preferences and the Value of Children

Ideal and Desired Family Size

Not only do the Southern Thai Muslims and the Thai Muslims have a greater number of live births, they also report wanting a larger ideal and desired family size than the Chinese and the Thais. The data also show that the urban respondents of all ethnic groups want a smaller ideal and desired family size than their rural counterparts. It is also interesting to note that wives of all ethnic groups want a smaller ideal and desired family size than their husbands. The average ideal family size of the rural Southern Thai Muslims, the rural Thai Muslims, the rural Chinese and the rural Thais is 3.75, 3.35, 3.35 and 2.90 respectively, and their respective urban ideal family size is 3.44, 3.17, 3.21 and 2.70. The mean ideal number of sons of all ethnic groups is greater than that of daughters.

As for additional number of children desired by the respondents, the Southern Thai Muslims still average the greatest number, followed by the Thai Muslims, the Chinese and the Thais. It is interesting to note that the respondents report that their spouse desired a greater additional number of children than themselves.

Sex Preference

All ethnic groups express preference for sons to daughters as indicated by a difference between mean ideal number of sons compared to that of daughters. The former is consistently greater than the latter.

The respondents were also asked if they were to have exactly three children only, how many sons would they like to have. In this case, all ethnic groups still show a bias in favour of sons. This bias is most apparent among the Chinese, followed by the Thai Muslims, the Southern Thai Muslims and the Thais, respectively.

The findings show significant differences among the ethnic groups in the level of fertility as measured by pregnancies, live births and birth intervals, and in the number of living children and children living away from home. The Southern Thai Muslims and the Thai Muslims have higher fertility than the Thais and the Chinese. The Thais average lower fertility than any other ethnic group. Fertility is also higher among the rural members of all ethnic groups than their urban counterparts. The Thais also express a desire for a smaller ideal and desired family size and less preference for sons than any other ethnic group.

Differences in Family Planning

Knowledge of Birth Control

The survey also collected data on knowledge, attitudes and birth control practices of all ethnic groups. The data show that the Thais are better informed on birth control than the Chinese, the Thai Muslims and the Southern Thai Muslims, respectively. The percentages of the rural members of the ethnic groups who have heard of birth control are 92 per cent for the Thais, 88 per cent for the Chinese, 87 per cent for the Thai Muslims and 65 per cent for the Southern Thai Muslims (Table 4.2). In general, more urban respondents have heard of family planning members. The Thais, the Chinese and the Thai Muslim men in rural areas are better informed than their wives. The exception are the Southern Thai Muslim men who are less informed of birth control than their women. Their ignorance and resultant attitudes can be a hindrance to the group's adoption of birth control. The data suggest that there is a real need to conduct family planning campaigns among the Southern Thai Muslims. The Southern Thai Muslim men should be better informed than they are now.

Current and Future Use of Contraception

The percentage of respondents currently using birth control is consistently lowest among the Southern Thai Muslims (22 per cent in the rural and 27 per cent in the urban areas), highest among the Thais (56 per cent in the rural and 59 per cent in the urban areas). Among the Chinese, 45 per cent of the rural and 57 per cent of the urban women are currently practising birth control, and among the Thai Muslims, 40.3 per cent of the rural and 48 per cent of the urban women are currently practising family planning. A similar pattern of differences among the ethnic groups are also found for the category of respondents who have ever used contraception.

The relative lack of contraceptive knowledge among the Southern Thai Muslim men and women results in a low current usage of contraception as well as a low intent in future use. Only 8 per cent of the rural and 16 per cent of the urban Southern Thai Muslim women plan to use birth control as compared to 58 per cent of the rural and 51 per cent of the urban Thai women, and half of the rural and urban Chinese. Among the Thai Muslims, 52 per cent of the rural and 57 per cent in the urban female population express interest in using birth control in the future. The opportunity for increasing family planning practices among the Thai Muslims, the Chinese and the Thais are more encouraging than among the Southern Thai Muslims.

Methods Currently Used

The most frequently used contraceptive method among all ethnic groups is the pill: 53.5 per cent and 48.5 per cent of the rural and urban Thai women, 50.0 per cent and 37.4 per cent of the rural and urban Thai Muslim women, 46.1 per cent and 43.5 per cent of the rural and urban Chinese, and 45.2 per cent and 57.8 per cent of the rural and urban Southern Thai Muslims, respectively.

The second most frequently used method varies by ethnic group: the condom is preferred among the Chinese; female sterilization among the Thais; injectables among the Thai Muslims; and the IUD among the urban Southern Thai Muslims. The third frequently used method also varies by ethnic group: it is

TABLE 4.2
Birth Control by Ethnic Group

Variable	Chinese Rural Female	Chinese Rural Male	Chinese Urban Female	Chinese Urban Male	Thai Rural Female	Thai Rural Male	Thai Urban Female	Thai Urban Male
Percentage Who Have Heard of Birth Control	88.3	93.2	93.4	91.4	91.6	92.7	94.7	91.0
Percentage Currently Using Birth Control	44.5	52.9	56.5	65.8	55.7	53.5	58.7	60.0
Percentage of All Respondents Who Have Ever Used Contraception	73.4	80.5	77.7	76.7	75.0	77.3	77.0	86.6
Percentage of Current Non-Users Who Plan to Use in the Future	50.0	53.8	48.8	64.0	57.6	42.3	50.6	73.7
Percentage of Current Users Using Each Method								
1 = Pill	46.1	37.1	43.5	37.5	53.5	49.1	48.5	33.3
2 = IUD	9.0	5.7	6.5	10.4	8.5	5.7	5.9	6.7
3 = Diaphram	1.1	-	-	-	-	-	-	-
4 = Foam, jelly, cream	-	-	-	-	-	-	0.7	2.2
5 = Douche	-	-	-	-	-	-	1.5	-
6 = Condom	23.6	28.6	15.7	20.8	3.9	9.4	12.5	15.6
7 = Rhythm	7.9	11.4	12.0	8.3	1.6	1.9	3.7	2.2
8 = Withdrawal	-	-	-	-	0.8	1.9	-	-
9 = Abstention	-	-	-	-	-	-	-	-
10 = Female sterilization	6.7	14.3	13.1	14.6	21.7	17.0	14.0	28.9
11 = Male sterilization	-	-	0.9	-	1.6	7.5	5.9	4.4
12 = Injectables	5.6	2.9	8.3	8.4	8.4	7.5	6.6	6.7
13 = Others	-	-	-	-	-	-	0.7	-
Total	100.0	100.0	100.0	100.0	100.0	100.0	100.0	100.0

TABLE 4.2 (cont'd)

Variable	Thai Muslim				Southern Thai Muslim			
	Rural		Urban		Rural		Urban	
	Female	Male	Female	Male	Female	Male	Female	Male
Percentage Who Have Heard of Birth Control	87.5	91.8	91.3	85.2	65.6	60.4	75.3	68.8
Percentage Currently Using Birth Control	40.3	50.0	48.4	45.9	22.3	19.6	27.1	20.7
Percentage of All Respondents Who Have Ever Used Contraception	57.6	65.1	71.0	62.6	27.2	25.0	31.7	22.0
Percentage of Current Non-Users Who Plan to Use in the Future	51.7	46.8	56.9	42.5	8.3	6.4	15.9	14.5
Percentage of Current Users Using Each Method								
1 = Pill	50.5	52.3	37.4	25.0	45.2	50.0	57.8	35.3
2 = IUD	3.1	4.5	8.4	12.5	9.5	15.0	17.8	17.6
3 = Diaphram	-	-	0.9	-	-	-	-	-
4 = Foam, jelly, cream	-	-	-	-	-	-	-	-
5 = Douche	-	-	-	-	-	-	-	-
6 = Condom	2.1	11.4	8.5	25.0	-	15.0	4.4	29.4
7 = Rhythm	5.2	6.8	12.1	25.0	14.4	-	2.2	5.9
8 = Withdrawal	-	-	-	-	-	-	-	-
9 = Abstention	-	-	-	-	-	-	-	-
10 = Female sterilization	15.4	13.6	14.0	3.1	11.9	10.0	6.7	5.9
11 = Male sterilization	1.0	2.3	4.7	3.1	-	-	-	-
12 = Injectables	22.7	9.1	13.1	6.3	19.0	10.0	8.9	-
13 = Others	-	-	0.9	-	-	-	2.2	5.9
Total	100.0	100.0	100.0	100.0	100.0	100.0	100.0	100.0

TABLE 4.2 (cont'd)
Birth Control by Ethnic Group

Variable	Chinese				Thai			
	Rural		Urban		Rural		Urban	
	Female	Male	Female	Male	Female	Male	Female	Male
Satisfaction with Method among Current Users								
3 = Very satisfied	64.8	66.7	54.7	39.1	65.3	69.2	62.4	52.5
2 = Fairly satisfied	28.4	33.3	42.5	52.2	28.8	25.6	30.4	42.5
1 = Dissatisfied	6.8	-	2.8	8.7	5.9	5.2	7.2	5.0
Total	100.0	100.0	100.0	100.0	100.0	100.0	100.0	100.0
Birth Control Intentions of Current Users								
1 = Continue method	82.4	84.8	82.2	82.6	80.3	76.3	78.4	78.1
2 = Change method	14.1	12.1	16.9	17.4	18.8	23.7	19.2	19.5
3 = Stop	3.5	3.1	0.9	-	0.9	-	2.4	2.4
Total	100.0	100.0	100.0	100.0	100.0	100.0	100.0	100.0

TABLE 4.2 (cont'd)

Variable	Thai Muslim				Southern Thai Muslim			
	Rural		Urban		Rural		Urban	
	Female	Male	Female	Male	Female	Male	Female	Male
Satisfaction with Method among Current Users								
3 = Very satisfied	68.4	57.8	62.5	50.0	62.5	68.4	47.7	64.7
2 = Fairly satisfied	28.4	40.0	30.8	46.9	32.5	31.6	50.0	35.3
1 = Dissatisfied	3.2	2.2	6.7	3.1	5.0	-	2.3	-
Total	100.0	100.0	100.0	100.0	100.0	100.0	100.0	100.0
Birth Control Intentions of Current Users								
1 = Continue method	74.7	76.1	71.3	65.6	66.7	73.7	84.1	70.6
2 = Change method	22.1	15.2	22.8	28.1	20.5	21.1	11.4	17.6
3 = Stop	3.2	8.7	5.9	6.3	12.8	5.2	4.5	11.8
Total	100.0	100.0	100.0	100.0	100.0	100.0	100.0	100.0

the IUD among the rural Chinese; female sterilization among the urban Chinese; female sterilization among the rural and urban Thai Muslims; and the rhythm method among the urban Southern Thai Muslims. It is obvious that the methods used by the Southern Thai Muslims are in general less effective than those used by other ethnic groups. This is consistent with their lack of contraceptive knowledge.

Satisfaction with Current Methods

It is noteworthy that the great majority of current users of all ethnic groups are satisfied with the method(s) they currently use. Over 60 per cent of the Thai, the Chinese and the Thai Muslim and the rural Southern Thai Muslims say they are very satisfied with the method(s) they currently use. The great majority of them, over 70 per cent, also intend to continue using the method(s). However, the percentage of respondents who want to change method(s) is relatively high among the Thai Muslims, the Southern Thai Muslims, perhaps because the methods that they are using are not as effective as they would like them to be.

Accessibility of Birth Control

The difference in knowledge and practice of contraception among the four ethnic groups corresponds with the ease of accessibility of birth control. Over three-fourths of the Thai and the Chinese respondents, compared with about 65 per cent of the Thai Muslims and one-fourth of the Southern Thai Muslims, know where to get birth control information or supplies (Table 4.3). Lack of information or knowledge of where to obtain such information is one great stumbling block to greater participation in family planning especially among the Southern Thai Muslims.

The mean distance to the sources is reported ranging from 13 minutes among the urban Chinese to 36 minutes among the rural Thai Muslims. The Thai Muslims in all parts of the country have to spend a longer time getting to family planning services. This is consistent with their low percentage of contraceptive use. Low use may also be due to the fact that they do not want their neighbours to know that they practice family planning as it is against their religious norms.

Cost and Difficulties in Getting Supply

The cost of getting a one-month supply of contraceptives varies by ethnic groups as different groups favour different combinations of contraceptive methods. The average cost ranges from about Bht 22 to Bht 118 a month. The urban Thais and urban Chinese give a lower cost than their rural counterparts.

In addition to financial cost, the respondents also express other difficulties associated with family planning. These include embarrassment, the dissatisfaction with medical personnel in the family planning clinics, (attitudes, different ethnicity, etc.), distance or transportation problems, childcare worries and others. Among the Thai Muslims, the problems with medical personnel, distance and childcare problems predominate. Among the Thais and the Chinese, distance and childcare are major problems.

Attitudes Towards Birth Control and Liked and Disliked Characteristics of Methods

The data on attitudes towards birth control show that the Thai and the Chinese approve the use of birth control among married couples more than the Thai Muslims and the Southern Thai Muslims (Table 4.4).

Regarding method characteristic(s), the majority dislike contraceptive methods that may affect health and methods that are unpleasant to use. The Southern Thai Muslims and the Thai Muslims are more concerned with irreversibility of contraception than the Thais and the Chinese. The Thais and the Chinese are also less concerned with the methods that require examination of the wife by a man or surgery than the Thai Muslims and the Southern Thai Muslims. Obviously, the Muslim people dislike methods that are against their own religion more than the Thais and the Chinese.

As for the liked characteristic(s) of contraceptive methods, the data show the majority of the Thais and the Chinese like methods that are convenient to use, very effective, permanent and easily controlled by self. It is interesting to note that more than half of the Southern Thai Muslims consistently do not accept any of the "liked characteristics" of the methods.

Approval of abortion is highest if the pregnancy seriously endangers the woman's life. The Southern Thai Muslims and the Thai Muslims are still more conservative than the Thais and the Chinese. Approval is somewhat less in the situation where the family cannot afford another child and considerably less or even rejected in the situation where the woman prefers to have her child at a later date. The Thais are least conservative in this respect.

TABLE 4.3
Accessibility of Birth Control by Ethnic Group

	Chinese				Thai			
	Rural		Urban		Rural		Urban	
Variable	Female	Male	Female	Male	Female	Male	Female	Male
Percentage Who Know Where to Get Information or Supplies	82.1	73.6	83.2	76.2	85.0	78.2	83.9	78.4
Distance to Source in Minutes	30.52	21.12	14.81	13.69	26.24	17.46	19.07	18.55
(Mean, Standard Deviation)	45.57	19.79	16.53	15.92	49.69	15.54	27.30	30.47
Expected Cost of One-Month Supply	117.70	116.58	73.63	92.06	45.18	29.00	41.54	22.88
(Mean, Standard Deviation)	234.68	211.57	140.84	160.57	107.52	53.91	97.14	48.08
Difficulties in Obtaining Method, Aside from Cost								
0 = No difficulties	94.0	92.3	95.8	93.3	83.8	91.2	88.4	94.9
1 = Embarrassment	0.7	-	-	-	-	-	-	-
2 = Medical personnel (attitudes, different ethnicity, etc.)	2.0	-	-	-	0.8	-	0.6	2.6

TABLE 4.3 (cont'd)

Variable	Thai Muslim				Southern Thai Muslim			
	Rural		Urban		Rural		Urban	
	Female	Male	Female	Male	Female	Male	Female	Male
Percentage Who Know Where to Get Information or Supplies	73.6	64.5	79.5	72.1	51.8	61.0	62.1	63.2
Distance to Source in Minutes	26.08	35.92	23.35	33.12	25.06	23.31	26.46	32.26
(Mean, Standard Deviation)	27.74	76.23	49.71	120.17	26.59	28.50	33.21	42.58
Expected Cost of One-Month Supply	41.16	55.64	93.91	67.18	22.43	65.46	35.65	36.00
(Mean, Standard Deviation)	84.74	150.98	181.18	172.03	54.48	160.59	59.90	79.29
Difficulties in Obtaining Method, Aside from Cost								
0 = No difficulties	85.1	84.8	86.5	85.0	81.4	90.6	85.2	92.0
1 = Embarrassment	-	2.2	-	-	-	-	3.6	-
2 = Medical personnel (attitudes, different ethnicity, etc.)	3.1	2.2	1.5	-	-	-	-	-

TABLE 4.3 (cont'd)
Accessibility of Birth Control by Ethnic Group

	Chinese				Thai			
	Rural		Urban		Rural		Urban	
Variable	Female	Male	Female	Male	Female	Male	Female	Male
Difficulties in Obtaining Method, Aside from Cost								
3 = Distance or transportation	-	2.5	0.7	-	2.9	-	-	-
4 = Childcare	-	2.6	1.4	-	1.5	-	4.3	-
5 = Other	3.3	2.6	2.1	6.7	11.0	8.8	6.7	2.5
Total	100.0	100.0	100.0	100.0	100.0	100.0	100.0	100.0

TABLE 4.3 (cont'd)

Variable	Thai Muslim				Southern Thai Muslim			
	Rural		Urban		Rural		Urban	
	Female	Male	Female	Male	Female	Male	Female	Male
Difficulties in Obtaining Method, Aside from Cost								
3 = Distance or transportation	0.8	-	-	-	4.7	-	1.9	-
4 = Childcare	5.5	-	3.7	5.0	2.3	-	1.9	-
5 = Other	5.5	10.8	8.3	10.0	11.6	9.4	7.4	8.0
Total	100.0	100.0	100.0	100.0	100.0	100.0	100.0	100.0

TABLE 4.4
Attitudes towards Birth Control and Liked and Disliked
Characteristics of Birth Control Method(s) by Ethnic Group

Variable	Chinese				Thai			
	Rural		Urban		Rural		Urban	
	Female	Male	Female	Male	Female	Male	Female	Male
Approval of Married Couples								
Using Birth Control	3.93	4.01	3.95	4.03	3.99	2.89	4.07	4.08
(Mean, Standard Deviation)	0.99	0.81	0.86	0.87	1.03	1.07	0.94	0.90
Percentage Who Consider "Very Important" Each Disliked Method Characteristic								
May affect health	77.9	73.6	82.6	87.6	82.6	81.8	85.1	79.4
Unpleasant to use	61.6	52.8	63.7	54.3	60.7	57.3	57.6	57.8
Irreversible	38.6	34.3	34.1	42.9	45.7	44.0	37.2	43.1
Requires examination of wife by a man	17.0	11.3	16.4	17.1	23.5	15.6	16.4	17.6
Requires surgery	28.0	18.9	30.3	21.9	36.2	30.9	27.9	26.5
Against own religion	17.6	14.2	20.3	9.6	26.1	24.5	24.1	16.7
Percentage Who Consider "Very Important" Each Liked Method Characteristic								
Convenient to use	69.3	77.4	76.1	68.3	78.5	77.3	74.8	75.2
Very effective	72.9	77.4	74.0	66.3	72.0	63.6	71.7	67.3
Permanent	60.8	62.3	56.9	51.0	64.5	49.1	56.5	51.5
Easily controlled by self	66.3	67.9	59.9	47.6	58.4	52.3	53.4	50.5

TABLE 4.4 (cont'd)

Variable	Thai Muslim				Southern Thai Muslim			
	Rural		Urban		Rural		Urban	
	Female	Male	Female	Male	Female	Male	Female	Male
Approval of Married Couples								
Using Birth Control	3.75	3.60	3.69	3.42	3.21	3.27	3.30	3.10
(Mean, Standard Deviation)	1.14	1.17	1.13	1.29	1.19	1.11	1.04	1.08
Percentage Who Consider								
"Very Important" Each								
Disliked Method Characteristic								
May affect health	82.7	81.8	82.7	86.5	71.9	66.3	73.2	55.3
Unpleasant to use	63.4	60.9	60.7	56.8	54.1	55.4	46.0	52.1
Irreversible	49.5	55.0	50.9	52.3	61.9	62.4	60.3	61.7
Requires examination of								
wife by a man	30.2	19.3	28.9	30.6	50.3	47.5	42.6	50.0
Requires surgery	45.1	34.5	40.8	34.2	68.5	72.3	54.5	55.3
Against own religion	55.3	64.0	46.9	47.7	81.7	84.2	83.2	80.9
Percentage Who Consider								
"Very Important" Each								
Liked Method Characteristic								
Convenient to use	72.4	73.6	71.9	70.3	43.1	45.0	45.0	41.5
Very effective	72.4	66.4	68.5	63.1	44.2	36.0	43.9	42.6
Permanent	51.2	42.7	56.5	47.3	38.1	31.3	36.5	41.5
Easily controlled by self	57.9	66.4	65.5	52.3	48.7	49.5	47.1	47.9

TABLE 4.4 (cont'd)
Attitudes towards Birth Control and Liked and Disliked
Characteristics of Birth Control Method(s) by Ethnic Group

Variable	Chinese				Thai			
	Rural		Urban		Rural		Urban	
	Female	Male	Female	Male	Female	Male	Female	Male
Approval of Abortion Under Different Conditions (Mean on 5-point Scale)								
If the pregnancy seriously endangers the woman's life	3.89	3.90	4.01	3.91	3.82	3.84	3.89	3.84
(Mean, Standard Deviation)	1.36	1.33	1.29	1.31	1.49	1.38	1.43	1.40
If the family cannot afford another child	2.33	2.32	2.46	2.60	2.50	2.48	2.62	2.38
(Mean, Standard Deviation)	1.39	1.35	1.41	1.38	1.48	1.32	1.40	1.33
If the woman prefers to have her child at a later date	1.79	1.76	1.99	2.24	2.01	2.02	2.06	2.07
(Mean, Standard Deviation)	1.07	0.97	1.12	1.18	1.26	1.15	1.15	1.13

TABLE 4.4 (cont'd)

Variable	Thai Muslim				Southern Thai Muslim			
	Rural		Urban		Rural		Urban	
	Female	Male	Female	Male	Female	Male	Female	Male
Approval of Abortion Under Different Conditions (Mean on 5-point Scale)								
If the pregnancy seriously endangers the woman's life	3.30	3.43	3.66	3.64	3.12	3.36	3.12	3.19
(Mean, Standard Deviation)	1.60	1.48	1.49	1.54	1.44	1.39	1.47	1.44
If the family cannot afford another child	1.96	1.98	2.07	1.91	2.43	2.58	2.40	2.59
(Mean, Standard Deviation)	1.23	1.06	1.36	1.26	1.23	1.20	1.29	1.26
If the woman prefers to have her child at a later date	1.71	1.68	1.70	1.62	2.37	2.40	2.27	2.53
(Mean, Standard Deviation)	1.08	1.07	1.14	0.93	1.22	1.19	1.21	1.28

Differences in Other Variables Affecting Fertility

In addition to knowledge, attitude towards and practice of contraception, there are other natural and socio-economic factors affecting fertility. The data show that more Thai Muslims and Southern Thai Muslims, who have had a larger family size, claim that it is physically possible for them to have another child than the Thais and the Chinese (Table 4.5). However, more Thai and Chinese women than the Thai Muslim women in the South and in other parts of the country consider it very easy for them to get pregnant. The Southern Thai Muslims who claim it is easy for them to get pregnant constitute less than one-fifth whereas about one-third of other ethnic groups make such a claim. Of all ethnic groups, fewer husbands than wives and more urban couples than the rural ones perceive that they are fecund.

Sexual Abstention and Breastfeeding

Regarding a desired period of abstention from sexual intercourse after birth, the Southern Thai Muslims gave the longest period, a minimum of 3.1 months, compared with 2.5, 2.7 and 2.9 months given by the Thais, Thai Muslims and Chinese in the rural areas.

Breastfeeding is fairly widespread among all the ethnic groups. More than 70 per cent of the respondents of each ethnic group have breastfed their most recent child. The data also show that the Chinese breastfeed for a shorter duration than any other group. This is followed by the Thais and the Thai Muslims. The rural Southern Thai Muslims report the longest breastfeeding period (11.5 months). The differences among the ethnic groups in the number of additional months of breastfeeding with supplement are similar to the differences in the duration of breastfeeding of the most recent child.

Value of Children

In Thai society, as in any other societies, children are regarded as assets as well as liabilities. The social and cultural characteristics of the ethnic groups significantly affect their assessment of advantages and disadvantages of having children (Table 4.6). About 45.6 per cent of the rural Southern Thai Muslims and the rural Thai Muslims stress children's help in old age as a major advantage of having children compared with 31 per cent of the Chinese and 29 per cent of the Thais. Other advantages of having children include family continuity, companionship and love, and a source of happiness. The Chinese and also the Thai Muslims stress family continuity as an advantage of having children more than the Thais and the Southern Thai Muslims.

The respondents were also directly asked whether they expect economic support from children in old age. The number of urban respondents who expect such support is lower than the rural respondents. Similarly, fewer men than women, except among the Southern Thai Muslim men, expect such support. As for the differences among the three ethnic groups, over 70 per cent of the Southern Thai Muslims expect major support from their children in old age. Only 44.2 per cent of the rural and 38.4 per cent of the Thai Muslims, compared with 47.4 per cent of the rural and 26.7 per cent of the urban Thais, expect major economic support from their children.

The great majority of the respondents from all ethnic groups expect that the life of their children will be better. Men have lower expectations than women, and urban people less than the rural ones. There are few differences among the ethnic groups in this respect.

Disadvantages of Having Children

As for disadvantages of having children, it is interesting to note that no less than one-third of the respondents from all ethnic groups consider cost of education and other financial costs of having children a major disadvantage (Table 4.7). Worry over the child's future is also considered a disadvantage by 10 per cent of the Chinese and 7 per cent of the Thai Muslims. Fewer Thais and Southern Thai Muslims regard this as a disadvantage. Restrictions on parents such as feeling tied down and inability to work are also stressed by 15 per cent of the rural and 26 per cent of the urban Southern Thai Muslims, 12 per cent of the rural Thais and 9 per cent of the urban Thais.

When asked whether they would be embarrassed at becoming pregnant when they already have grandchildren, over half of the rural Chinese and the rural Thais stated that they would be greatly embarrassed. In contrast only one-fifth of the Southern Thai Muslims said so. The urban and male respondents felt less embarrassed at having another child then than the rural and female respondents. Over 14 per cent the Thai Muslims, followed by 12 per cent the Southern Thai Muslims, 10 per cent the Chinese and the 7.1 per cent of the Thais say they would be happy in such a situation.

The extent to which having many children would impose

TABLE 4.5

Perceived Fecundity, Sexual Abstention and Breastfeeding by Ethnic Group

Variable	Chinese				Thai			
	Rural		Urban		Rural		Urban	
	Female	Male	Female	Male	Female	Male	Female	Male
Fecundity								
Physically possible for couple to have another child								
3 = Yes	51.0	47.2	51.7	62.4	54.3	50.0	53.4	52.6
2 = Don't know	10.6	7.9	8.2	4.3	5.4	6.6	6.4	4.0
1 = No	38.4	44.9	40.1	33.3	40.3	43.4	40.2	43.4
Total	100.0	100.0	100.0	100.0	100.0	100.0	100.0	100.0
Ease in Getting Pregnant								
4 = Very easy	31.1	27.9	26.5	22.2	35.5	32.0	30.8	34.7
3 = Fairly easy	35.7	39.4	37.9	43.4	35.0	40.8	38.1	36.7
2 = A little difficult	20.7	23.1	24.3	27.3	17.2	17.5	18.2	19.4
1 = Very difficult	12.2	9.6	11.3	7.1	12.3	9.7	12.9	9.2
0 = Not possible any longer	0.3	-	-	-	-	-	-	-
Total	100.0	100.0	100.0	100.0	100.0	100.0	100.0	100.0
Sexual Intercourse								
Desirable Abstention after Birth (Months)	2.88	2.55	2.38	2.87	2.50	2.74	2.39	2.83
(Mean, Standard Deviation)	4.20	2.38	1.22	3.71	1.31	2.41	1.04	3.79

TABLE 4.5 (cont'd)

Variable	Thai Muslim				Southern Thai Muslim			
	Rural		Urban		Rural		Urban	
	Female	Male	Female	Male	Female	Male	Female	Male
Fecundity								
Physically possible for couple to have another child								
3 = Yes	65.4	64.1	58.0	64.1	59.6	56.5	61.7	65.6
2 = Don't know	10.8	10.4	6.7	6.8	33.7	38.4	27.2	25.6
1 = No	23.8	25.5	53.3	29.1	6.7	5.1	11.1	8.8
Total	100.0	100.0	100.0	100.0	100.0	100.0	100.0	100.0
Ease in Getting Pregnant								
4 = Very easy	29.9	19.5	29.3	27.1	10.5	10.7	17.3	11.5
3 = Fairly easy	36.7	39.8	29.3	31.8	23.3	22.3	24.0	19.5
2 = A little difficult	21.7	13.5	27.3	19.6	56.1	47.9	44.7	54.0
1 = Very difficult	11.7	8.3	13.8	19.6	10.1	19.1	13.4	13.8
0 = Not possible any longer	-	0.9	0.3	1.9	-	-	0.6	1.2
Total	100.0	100.0	100.0	100.0	100.0	100.0	100.0	100.0
Sexual Intercourse								
Desirable Abstention after Birth (Months)	2.67	3.62	2.86	2.84	3.11	3.17	3.08	3.06
(Mean, Standard Deviation)	1.84	9.52	4.73	3.96	1.65	1.78	3.20	4.05

TABLE 4.5 (cont'd)

Perceived Fecundity, Sexual Abstention and Breastfeeding by Ethnic Group

Variable	Chinese				Thai			
	Rural		Urban		Rural		Urban	
	Female	Male	Female	Male	Female	Male	Female	Male
Breastfeeding								
Percentage breastfed most recent child	76.1	87.5	72.3	77.8	82.7	70.0	75.7	53.3
Months of Full Breastfeeding	7.15	-	5.06	-	8.84	-	6.02	-
(Mean Among Those Who Breastfed, Standard Deviation)	9.38	-	5.91	-	8.50	-	7.69	-
Additional Months of Breastfeeding with Supplement	4.44	0.32	3.14	0.17	6.09	1.01	3.92	0.66
(Mean Among Those Who Breastfed, Standard Deviation)	7.18	1.72	4.70	0.84	7.57	6.00	6.50	4.44

TABLE 4.5 (cont'd)

Variable	Thai Muslim				Southern Thai Muslim			
	Rural		Urban		Rural		Urban	
	Female	Male	Female	Male	Female	Male	Female	Male
Breastfeeding								
Percentage breastfed most recent child	83.6	90.0	77.7	100.0	74.4	68.2	73.1	81.8
Months of Full Breastfeeding	8.64	-	6.21	-	11.49	-	8.54	-
(Mean Among Those Who Breastfed, Standard Deviation)	8.28	-	7.46	-	13.25	-	10.56	-
Additional Months of Breastfeeding with Supplement	6.14	1.09	3.97	-	8.44	1.41	5.89	1.38
(Mean Among Those Who Breastfed, Standard Deviation)	7.64	6.82	6.32	-	11.60	4.44	9.63	4.63

TABLE 4.6

Value of Children by Ethnic Group

Variable	Chinese				Thai			
	Rural		Urban		Rural		Urban	
	Female	Male	Female	Male	Female	Male	Female	Male
Advantages of Having Children								
Help in housework	3.8	5.1	3.7	3.1	4.5	2.1	3.1	2.0
Help in old age	30.9	25.6	22.8	13.5	29.0	29.5	24.4	24.5
Financial, practical help	3.1	1.3	2.5	5.0	8.6	4.9	4.2	3.9
Family name, line	21.8	31.2	14.5	34.5	7.6	16.8	8.6	18.6
Religion, social obligations	-	-	-	-	-	-	-	-
Adult status, social norms	-	-	-	1.2	0.9	-	0.9	-
Rewarding interactions	-	-	-	-	-	-	0.5	-
Companionship, love	21.5	17.2	28.8	14.5	20.0	12.1	22.8	22.5
Happiness	6.7	9.7	11.3	14.5	12.0	14.0	17.5	10.8
Play, fun, distraction	7.1	6.0	6.2	5.9	7.6	4.9	9.2	6.9
Martial bond	1.2	1.3	4.9	2.1	2.7	6.8	5.5	6.8
Psychological appreciation	0.9	-	2.1	1.2	1.5	-	0.6	1.0
Living through children	0.6	1.3	0.6	-	0.5	-	-	1.0
Achievement, power	-	-	-	1.2	-	-	0.8	-
Character, responsibility, incentive to succeed	-	1.3	1.1	-	-	1.2	0.6	2.0
Fulfillment	0.5	-	0.9	2.1	1.2	-	0.8	-
Other	1.9	-	0.6	1.2	3.9	7.7	0.5	-
Total	100.0	100.0	100.0	100.0	100.0	100.0	100.0	100.0

TABLE 4.6 (cont'd)

Variable	Thai Muslim				Southern Thai Muslim			
	Rural		Urban		Rural		Urban	
	Female	Male	Female	Male	Female	Male	Female	Male
Advantages of Having Children								
Help in housework	6.9	0.9	3.3	5.4	3.9	4.3	12.7	1.5
Help in old age	44.6	41.2	30.3	26.2	45.6	64.6	41.7	46.2
Financial, practical help	1.9	2.8	4.3	0.9	9.5	2.3	3.8	8.7
Family name, line	14.0	26.9	17.1	26.1	5.9	7.1	1.9	8.7
Religion, social obligations	0.5	-	-	-	-	-	-	-
Adult status, social norms	-	-	-	-	1.4	-	-	-
Rewarding interactions	-	-	-	-	0.8	-	-	-
Companionship, love	16.4	12.5	22.8	22.5	8.5	5.3	12.6	7.8
Happiness	7.9	8.9	10.8	8.1	18.1	15.1	19.4	15.0
Play, fun, distraction	3.6	1.9	5.5	0.9	5.5	-	2.4	1.4
Martial bond	-	-	2.1	2.7	-	-	2.9	5.7
Psychological appreciation	0.5	1.0	1.0	1.8	0.8	1.3	1.3	3.6
Living through children	0.5	1.0	-	-	-	-	-	-
Achievement, power	0.5	-	0.5	-	-	-	-	1.4
Character, responsibility, incentive to succeed	-	1.0	-	-	-	-	-	-
Fulfillment	1.2	-	0.8	3.6	-	-	-	-
Other	1.5	1.9	1.5	1.8	-	-	1.3	-
Total	100.0	100.0	100.0	100.0	100.0	100.0	100.0	100.0

TABLE 4.6 (cont'd)
Value of Children by Ethnic Group

Variable	Chinese				Thai			
	Rural		Urban		Rural		Urban	
	Female	Male	Female	Male	Female	Male	Female	Male
Expected Economic Support from Children in Old Age								
2 = Major	30.2	31.7	26.3	23.6	47.4	31.2	26.7	24.8
1 = Minor	36.5	28.8	35.4	36.0	26.3	31.2	29.7	27.7
0 = None	33.3	39.5	38.3	40.4	26.3	37.6	43.6	47.5
Total	100.0	100.0	100.0	100.0	100.0	100.0	100.0	100.0
Expectation About Life for Children								
3 = Better	91.8	89.4	87.9	82.7	93.4	95.5	83.5	83.3
2 = The same	5.6	8.7	7.6	7.7	5.0	4.5	10.9	10.8
1 = Worse	2.6	1.9	4.5	9.6	1.6	-	5.6	5.9
Total	100.0	100.0	100.0	100.0	100.0	100.0	100.0	100.0

TABLE 4.6 (cont'd)

Variable	Thai Muslim				Southern Thai Muslim			
	Rural		Urban		Rural		Urban	
	Female	Male	Female	Male	Female	Male	Female	Male
Expected Economic Support from Children in Old Age								
2 = Major	44.2	33.1	38.4	37.4	80.4	93.0	71.6	81.0
1 = Minor	38.3	35.8	37.7	40.4	8.2	3.0	9.5	4.3
0 = None	17.5	31.1	23.9	22.2	11.4	4.0	18.9	13.8
Total	100.0	100.0	100.0	100.0	100.0	100.0	100.0	100.0
Expectation About Life for Children								
3 = Better	91.8	86.6	89.8	91.7	92.3	95.0	89.6	90.6
2 = The same	6.8	8.9	7.3	5.5	7.7	4.0	7.8	9.4
1 = Worse	1.4	4.5	2.9	2.8	-	1.0	2.6	-
Total	100.0	100.0	100.0	100.0	100.0	100.0	100.0	100.0

TABLE 4.7
Disadvantages of Having Children

Variable	Chinese				Thai			
	Rural		Urban		Rural		Urban	
	Female	Male	Female	Male	Female	Male	Female	Male
Disadvantages of Having Children								
Financial costs								
Cost of education	16.9	27.9	3.2	14.1	1.6	3.7	3.6	5.3
Other financial costs	25.6	26.5	41.2	47.9	38.0	39.0	31.6	47.4
Childbearing Demands								
Physical stress	8.2	5.9	6.3	1.4	6.2	-	3.6	-
Emotional strain	5.9	5.9	8.1	1.4	5.0	2.4	9.1	-
Health, pregnancy	-	-	-	-	0.4	-	-	-
Discipline	1.8	4.4	3.6	2.8	2.3	1.2	1.6	-
Child's sickness	2.3	4.4	1.4	1.4	-	1.2	1.2	1.3
Worry over child's future	10.5	14.7	9.5	8.5	4.7	3.7	6.3	5.3
Other childbearing problems	0.9	-	2.3	8.5	1.6	-	0.4	-
Restrictions on Parents								
Tied down	3.2	2.9	4.5	-	7.4	1.2	3.6	-
Can't work	2.3	2.9	3.6	1.4	5.4	-	5.9	-

TABLE 4.7 (cont'd)

Variable	Thai Muslim				Southern Thai Muslim			
	Rural		Urban		Rural		Urban	
	Female	Male	Female	Male	Female	Male	Female	Male
sadvantages of Having Idren								
inancial costs								
ost of education	15.6	26.8	6.7	10.1	4.9	6.4	4.2	6.1
)ther financial costs	26.4	41.5	29.7	50.6	29.4	19.2	38.9	33.3
Idbearing Demands								
hysical stress	5.6	2.4	7.9	3.8	-	-	2.1	-
motional strain	3.9	-	6.7	2.5	6.1	6.4	2.1	-
lealth, pregnancy	-	-	-	-	-	-	0.7	-
)iscipline	4.3	2.4	6.3	6.3	-	-	0.7	-
hild's sickness	3.0	2.4	2.9	1.3	1.8	2.6	-	-
lorry over child's future	7.4	4.9	6.7	10.1	4.3	9.0	0.7	1.5
)ther childbearing problems	6.5	3.7	6.7	3.8	1.2	-	2.8	4.5
strictions on Parents								
ied down	5.2	3.7	2.9	-	7.4	12.8	18.1	10.6
an't work	3.5	1.2	0.4	2.5	7.4	11.5	9.7	4.5

TABLE 4.7 (cont'd)
Value of Children by Ethnic Group

Variable	Chinese				Thai			
	Rural		Urban		Rural		Urban	
	Female	Male	Female	Male	Female	Male	Female	Male
Cost of Social Relationship								
Marital strains	-	-	-	-	-	-	-	1.3
Social issues	-	-	-	-	0.4	-	0.8	-
Overpopulation	-	-	-	-	-	-	-	-
Miscellaneous	22.4	4.5	16.3	12.6	27.1	47.6	32.3	39.4
Total	100.0	100.0	100.0	100.0	100.0	100.0	100.0	100.0
Embarrassment at Becoming Pregnant after Having Grandchildren								
4 = Great embarrassment	53.8	43.8	46.5	27.7	52.5	46.8	53.0	37.0
3 = Mild embarrassment	13.5	12.4	18.5	18.8	14.3	14.7	13.2	12.0
2 = Indifference	22.5	23.8	23.9	34.7	26.1	33.0	24.0	33.0
1 = Happiness	10.2	20.0	11.1	18.8	7.1	5.5	9.8	18.0
Total	100.0	100.0	100.0	100.0	100.0	100.0	100.0	100.0

TABLE 4.7 (cont'd)

Variable	Thai Muslim				Southern Thai Muslim			
	Rural		Urban		Rural		Urban	
	Female	Male	Female	Male	Female	Male	Female	Male
ost of Social elationship								
Marital strains	-	-	-	-	-	1.3	0.7	-
Social issues	-	-	-	-	-	1.3	-	1.6
Overpopulation	-	-	-	-	-	-	-	-
Miscellaneous	18.6	11.0	23.1	8.8	37.5	29.5	19.3	37.9
Total	100.0	100.0	100.0	100.0	100.0	100.0	100.0	100.0
mbarrassment at ecoming Pregnant fter Having randchildren								
4 = Great embarrassment	45.1	26.8	52.2	30.0	19.0	20.0	20.9	11.5
3 = Mild embarrassment	14.8	20.5	10.8	17.2	22.5	37.0	28.3	32.2
2 = Indifference	26.6	28.6	23.1	37.3	46.7	32.0	40.3	44.8
1 = Happiness	13.5	24.1	13.9	15.5	11.8	11.0	10.5	11.5
Total	100.0	100.0	100.0	100.0	100.0	100.0	100.0	100.0

TABLE 4.7 (cont'd)
Value of Children by Ethnic Group

Variable	Chinese				Thai			
	Rural		Urban		Rural		Urban	
	Female	Male	Female	Male	Female	Male	Female	Male
Restrictions on Freedom to Enjoy Other Things from Many Children								
3 = A lot	12.8	7.4	15.8	9.5	24.4	8.1	17.7	8.9
2 = A little	41.3	42.1	38.8	37.1	40.6	45.5	39.4	43.1
1 = None	45.9	50.5	45.4	53.3	35.0	46.4	42.9	48.0
Total	100.0	100.0	100.0	100.0	100.0	100.0	100.0	100.0
What Children Prevent One from Enjoying								
Freedom and time								
Tied down; not free	26.2	19.3	34.4	25.9	28.9	25.8	24.7	28.4
Can't attend to own desires	14.5	22.0	15.2	22.1	13.3	13.9	12.1	14.8
Consumption Activities								
Must watch spending	9.1	15.6	9.3	-	8.9	13.0	8.0	15.7
Can't travel	17.4	22.0	13.3	17.3	15.0	16.7	15.5	19.6
Work Activities								
Can't work	14.5	21.1	16.4	17.4	24.4	18.5	23.2	21.5
Miscellaneous								
Less time with spouse	8.7	-	-	-	-	-	8.1	-
Other	9.6	-	11.4	17.3	9.5	12.1	8.4	-
Total	100.0	100.0	100.0	100.0	100.0	100.0	100.0	100.0

TABLE 4.7 (cont'd)

Variable	Thai Muslim				Southern Thai Muslim			
	Rural		Urban		Rural		Urban	
	Female	Male	Female	Male	Female	Male	Female	Male
estrictions on Freedom o Enjoy Other Things rom Many Children								
3 = A lot	16.8	13.4	17.0	5.4	7.6	11.0	12.4	7.3
2 = A little	33.7	32.1	33.3	28.8	44.4	46.0	46.1	32.3
1 = None	49.5	54.5	49.7	65.8	48.0	43.0	41.5	60.4
Total	100.0	100.0	100.0	100.0	100.0	100.0	100.0	100.0
nat Children Prevent ne from Enjoying								
Freedom and time								
Tied down; not free	26.6	23.9	26.2	19.5	26.9	24.6	32.7	25.8
Can't attend to own desires	24.2	21.2	15.5	15.1	15.8	11.7	16.7	15.4
onsumption Activities								
Must watch spending	-	-	9.3	11.5	-	12.7	8.9	13.4
Can't travel	16.2	22.1	12.1	15.9	15.2	15.7	11.5	13.4
ork Activities								
Can't work	18.8	16.8	14.6	15.0	28.9	22.6	19.7	18.6
iscellaneous								
Less time with spouse	-	-	8.7	11.5	-	-	-	-
Other	14.2	16.0	13.6	11.5	13.2	12.7	10.5	13.4
Total	100.0	100.0	100.0	100.0	100.0	100.0	100.0	100.0

restrictions on freedom to enjoy other things is also assessed differently by different ethnic groups. One-fourth of the rural and 18 per cent of the urban Thai women say that many children would impose a lot of restrictions on their freedom to enjoy other things, as compared to 16.8 per cent of the rural and 17.0 per cent of the urban Thai Muslims, 12.8 per cent of the rural and 16 per cent of the urban Chinese, and less than 10 per cent of the Southern Thai Muslims. Obviously, the Southern Thai Muslims feel less restricted at having many children than the Thai Muslims, the Chinese and the Thais.

When directly asked what children prevent one from enjoying, more than one-fourth of the respondents say they feel tied down and no longer have free time for themselves. A greater percentage of urban and female respondents than their rural and male counterparts felt this way. Slightly less than one-fourth of the respondents also say that children prevent them from working or from travelling. The differences among the ethnic groups in this respect are relatively small.

NUPTIALITY

Age at Marriage

As far as the marriage patterns and marriage attitudes among the respondents are concerned, the Southern Thai Muslims have the longest duration of marriage, about 12 years, due to their early age at marriage. A shorter duration is found among the Chinese, followed by the Thai Muslims and the Thais respectively. The Southern Thai Muslims women were married youngest, the average age being 17-18 years, compared with 20 and 21 for the rural and urban Thai Muslims and more than 21 for the Thai and the Chinese. The difference between the age of the husband and the wife is greatest among the Southern Thai Muslims, followed by the Thai Muslims, the Chinese and the Thais. The mean age of the husband at current marriage is 24 years for the Southern Thai Muslims, 26 years for the Thai Muslims and the Thais, and 27 years for the Chinese (Table 4.8).

For the great majority of the respondents, the current marriage is also their first marriage. The percentage of those who have had a previous marriage is highest among the Southern Thai Muslims, followed by the Thais, the Thai Muslims and the Chinese, respectively. Thus the age at first marriage of the great majority of the respondents of all ethnic groups is closest to the age at current marriage.

It is interesting but not surprising to note that the percentage of the respondents who are currently married to more than one spouse is highest among the Southern Thai Muslims, followed by the Thai Muslims, the Thais and the Chinese, respectively. However, the proportion involved in all cases is small. Less than 6 per cent of the Southern Thai Muslims, 2 per cent of the Thai Muslims and less than 1 per cent of the Thais are married to more than one spouse. This suggests that while polygamy is acceptable, especially for the Muslims it is not widely practised.

Death of spouse was reputedly the most common reason for those with at least one previous marriage. However, divorce or separation is highest among the Southern Thai Muslims. The data show that 8 per cent of previous marriages among the Southern Thai Muslims ended in divorce; less than 3 per cent among the Thais; and less than 1 per cent among the Thai Muslims. The Chinese marriage pattern is reportedly the most stable one.

Selection of the First Spouse

The four ethnic groups exhibit interesting differences in the patterns of mate selection. Over half of the Southern Thai Muslims' spouses were chosen for them by their parents or by their parents with their approval. In contrast, 80 per cent of the Thais, about 67 per cent of the Chinese, and 56 per cent of the Thai Muslims selected their own spouses or made the decision with the consent of their parents. Among the Thai Muslims, parents exercise the greatest control over the choice of the first spouse. This is followed by the Chinese and the Thais, respectively.

It is interesting to note that men are more self-reliant or independent than women, and the urban more than the rural respondents, in mate-selection.

Attitude Towards Celibacy

The respondents were asked to assess whether single or married women were better off. The majority of men from all ethnic groups agree that single women are worse off. However, less than half of the female respondents agree with the assessment. It is noteworthy that the percentage of the urban respondents who think that single women are worse off than married ones is less than that of the rural ones.

TABLE 4.8

Marriage and Marriage Attitudes by Ethnic Group

	Chinese				Thai			
	Rural		Urban		Rural		Urban	
Variable	Female	Male	Female	Male	Female	Male	Female	Male
Duration of Current Marriage	135.86	136.35	125.20	115.52	123.02	136.20	115.73	116.49
(Mean, Standard Deviation)	90.76	89.53	84.15	82.39	86.12	91.08	81.20	83.29
Age of Wife at Current Marriage	21.87	21.72	22.75	21.89	21.00	20.78	21.30	21.57
(Mean, Standard Deviation)	3.67	3.57	3.97	3.79	4.29	3.87	3.77	3.78
Age of Husband at Current Marriage	27.26	27.05	27.77	26.70	25.73	25.57	25.98	26.27
(Mean, Standard Deviation)	4.96	4.27	5.35	5.08	5.55	5.79	5.41	5.46
Previous Marriage								
1 = None	100.0	99.1	99.7	99.0	94.1	90.0	97.2	89.2
2 = One	-	0.9	0.3	1.0	5.3	7.3	2.8	6.9
3 = Two or more	-	-	-	-	0.6	2.7	-	3.9
Total	100.0	100.0	100.0	100.0	100.0	100.0	100.0	100.0
Percentage Currently Married to More than One Spouse	0.3	-	-	-	0.3	-	0.3	1.0

TABLE 4.8 (cont'd)

Variable	Thai Muslim				Southern Thai Muslim			
	Rural		Urban		Rural		Urban	
	Female	Male	Female	Male	Female	Male	Female	Male
Duration of Current Marriage	127.36	125.72	122.08	118.58	149.44	145.42	140.53	148.76
(Mean, Standard Deviation)	86.22	87.99	93.39	95.03	104.23	102.30	99.94	102.21
Age of Wife at Current								
Marriage	19.85	20.18	20.58	20.93	17.28	17.60	18.38	18.33
(Mean, Standard Deviation)	4.17	4.30	3.96	4.12	3.44	3.66	3.82	3.40
Age of Husband [a]at Current								
[m]Marriage	25.32	24.96	25.84	25.94	24.40	24.26	24.74	24.03
(Mean, Standard Deviation)	5.82	6.00	5.44	5.33	5.14	5.23	5.02	4.20
Previous Marriage								
1 = None	98.0	95.5	97.8	91.9	87.8	87.1	93.3	95.8
2 = One	2.0	3.6	2.2	7.2	8.6	9.9	5.7	4.2
3 = Two or more	-	0.9	-	0.9	3.6	3.0	1.0	-
Total	100.0	100.0	100.0	100.0	100.0	100.0	100.0	100.0
Percentage Currently Married								
to More than One Spouse	-	1.8	1.3	1.8	2.0	5.9	2.1	1.0

TABLE 4.8 (cont'd)
Marriage and Marriage Attitudes by Ethnic Group

Variable	Chinese				Thai			
	Rural		Urban		Rural		Urban	
	Female	Male	Female	Male	Female	Male	Female	Male
Age of R at First Marriage	21.83	26.82	22.76	26.37	20.66	24.15	21.15	25.01
(Mean, Standard Deviation)	3.86	4.08	4.36	5.09	4.16	5.52	3.86	5.25
Percentage of Respondents With at Least One Previous Marriage Ended By								
4 = Death	0.3	-	0.3	-	0.8	1.9	0.5	1.0
3 = Divorce	-	-	-	-	1.4	2.9	0.8	3.9
2 = Separation	-	-	-	-	0.9	1.1	-	-
1 = Married only once	99.7	100.0	99.7	100.0	96.9	94.1	98.7	95.1
Total	100.0	100.0	100.0	100.0	100.0	100.0	100.0	100.0
Who Decided on First Spouse								
1 = Parents	22.0	13.1	23.6	7.6	11.5	5.6	9.0	4.9
2 = Parents with R's approval	14.7	7.5	13.5	16.2	11.5	6.7	5.3	2.9
3 = Parents and R together	5.9	12.1	4.7	5.7	4.6	4.6	2.5	2.0
4 = R with parents' approval	22.5	16.8	27.7	21.0	23.8	14.8	29.6	16.7
5 = R	34.9	50.5	30.5	49.5	48.3	67.4	53.6	73.5
7 = Other	-	-	-	-	0.3	0.9	-	-
Total	100.0	100.0	100.0	100.0	100.0	100.0	100.0	100.0

TABLE 4.8 (cont'd)

Variable	Thai Muslim				Southern Thai Muslim			
	Rural		Urban		Rural		Urban	
	Female	Male	Female	Male	Female	Male	Female	Male
Age of R at First Marriage	19.67	23.97	20.58	25.34	17.05	22.48	17.85	23.09
(Mean, Standard Deviation)	3.78	5.32	3.95	5.18	4.47	5.83	4.47	5.45
Percentage of Respondents With at Least One Previous Marriage Ended By								
4 = Death	-	0.2	1.3	0.9	-	1.0	1.1	1.0
3 = Divorce	0.3	1.1	0.6	2.8	8.2	9.2	3.8	2.2
2 = Separation	0.3	-	0.3	3.7	-	-	0.8	1.0
1 = Married only once	99.4	98.7	97.8	92.6	91.8	89.8	94.3	95.8
Total	100.0	100.0	100.0	100.0	100.0	100.0	100.0	100.0
Who Decided on First Spouse								
1 = Parents	26.3	12.5	17.4	14.4	53.8	35.7	46.1	25.2
2 = Parents with R's approval	11.1	12.5	11.7	5.4	20.8	20.8	15.5	15.8
3 = Parents and R together	6.1	2.7	4.8	2.7	1.5	5.9	11.9	11.6
4 = R with parents' approval	20.2	15.1	23.9	20.7	10.2	19.8	4.7	11.7
5 = R	36.0	56.3	42.2	56.8	13.7	17.8	21.8	35.7
7 = Other	0.3	0.9	-	-	-	-	-	-
Total	100.0	100.0	100.0	100.0	100.0	100.0	100.0	100.0

TABLE 4.8 (cont'd)
Marriage and Marriage Attitudes by Ethnic Group

Variable	Chinese				Thai			
	Rural		Urban		Rural		Urban	
	Female	Male	Female	Male	Female	Male	Female	Male
Whether Single or Married Women are Better Off								
1 = Single are worse off	45.6	59.8	41.8	57.1	44.6	65.5	43.3	51.0
2 = Single are just as well off	23.1	25.2	29.6	26.7	20.4	12.7	19.2	28.4
3 = Single are better off	30.6	15.0	28.0	16.2	35.0	21.8	37.2	20.6
9 = Other	0.7	-	0.6	-	-	-	0.3	-
Total	100.0	100.0	100.0	100.0	100.0	100.0	100.0	100.0
Opinion on Polygamy								
3 = Approve	2.6	12.1	6.0	10.5	8.0	20.0	7.5	17.6
2 = Neutral	7.2	14.0	15.4	20.0	10.2	20.0	5.6	15.7
1 = Disapprove	88.2	68.2	76.1	64.7	79.9	59.1	85.4	62.8
9 = Other	2.0	5.6	2.5	4.8	1.9	0.9	1.5	3.9
Total	100.0	100.0	100.0	100.0	100.0	100.0	100.0	100.0

TABLE 4.8 (cont'd)

Variable	Thai Muslim				Southern Thai Muslim			
	Rural		Urban		Rural		Urban	
	Female	Male	Female	Male	Female	Male	Female	Male
Whether Single or Married Women are Better Off								
1 = Single are worse off	47.8	66.1	37.4	60.4	45.2	56.4	45.6	56.2
2 = Single are just as well off	18.5	15.2	24.2	22.5	41.1	34.7	41.5	34.4
3 = Single are better off	32.7	18.8	38.4	17.1	13.2	8.9	12.4	9.4
9 = Other	1.0	-	-	-	0.5	-	0.5	-
Total	100.0	100.0	100.0	100.0	100.0	100.0	100.0	100.0
Opinion on Polygamy								
3 = Approve	11.1	24.0	8.5	26.1	5.1	32.7	6.2	21.9
2 = Neutral	9.1	13.4	12.6	4.5	23.3	19.8	16.6	24.0
1 = Disapprove	79.1	56.3	75.8	58.6	71.6	46.5	77.2	52.1
9 = Other	0.7	6.3	3.1	10.8	-	1.0	-	2.0
Total	100.0	100.0	100.0	100.0	100.0	100.0	100.0	100.0

Polygamy

Regarding the respondents' opinion on polygamy, the majority of the respondents disapprove of polygamy except among the rural Southern Thai Muslims where polygamy is culturally and religiously acceptable. Not surprisingly, the percentage of the male respondents who approve of polygamy is higher than that of the female respondents. The percentage of approval of polygamy is highest among the Southern Thai Muslims, followed by the Thai Muslims, the Thais and the Chinese, respectively.

Divorce and Remarriage

With respect to grounds for divorce for women, the data show that the rural Thai males and the rural Thai Muslim males do not think that inability to have children is a condition for divorce. A greater percentage of the respondents from all ethnic groups also agree that cruelty to the wife and failure to support the family constitute grounds for divorce (Table 4.9).

It is interesting to note that the wife's desire to marry another man is not considered a condition for the wife to divorce her husband by the great majority of the respondents, except by a substantial proportion of the urban male respondents of all ethnic groups. In general, men are more liberal than women in approving divorce.

Widow Remarriage

The majority of the respondents from all ethnic groups approve of widow remarriage. However there are significant differences among them. The Thai Muslims have the greatest percentage approving widow remarriage, followed by the Thais, the Southern Thai Muslims, and the Chinese, respectively. Men are more liberal than women, and surprisingly, the rural respondents are more permissive than their urban counterparts.

The Thais and the Thai Muslims who are more liberal than the other two ethnic groups also approve widows remarrying at a higher mean age. The lowest mean age for approving widows remarrying is given by the Chinese.

Spouse Interaction

With respect to husband-wife interaction as measured by (1)

discussion about having another child, (2) sharing of worrries with spouse, and (3) whether spouse is chosen as the first or alternate person to spend leisure time with, the data show that over half of the respondents of all ethnic groups said they never discussed having another child. The percentage of affirmative responses is lowest among the Chinese, followed by the Southern Thai Muslims and the Thais. The percentage difference between the female rural and urban respondents is much less than among the male rural and urban respondents. In general the urban male respondents reported they discussed child-bearing matters with their spouse more than their rural counterparts (Table 4.10).

There are also significant ethnic differences in sharing of worries with spouse. Generally, the rural couples report a greater percentage of sharing than the urban ones, due to the fact that rural people probably spend more time with the family than their urban counterparts. The Thais share worries with the spouse more than the Thai Muslims, the Chinese and the Southern Thai Muslims, respectively.

Regarding whether the spouse is the person chosen to spend leisure time with, the great majority of the respondents responded in the affirmative. However, there are significant ethnic differences. The Thais report the highest percentage in choosing the spouse over another person to spend leisure time with, followed by the Chinese, the Southern Thai Muslims and the Thai Muslims. It is interesting to note that while the greater percentage of the Thais and the Chinese in urban areas chose their spouse to spend leisure time with than their rural counterparts, the opposite is true among the Thai Muslims and the Southern Thai Muslims. The finding implies either greater compatibility and equality among the Thai and Chinese urban couples than among the Muslim and the Southern Thai Muslim urban couples or greater multiple roles played by the wife in the urban Thai and Chinese families.

Women Status

On the perception of the role of women, two 5-point scale attitudes were used. A mean score of 2.5 is taken to be the neutral point and a higher score indicates stronger agreement. The two statements are "A girl becomes fully a woman only when she bears her own children" and "A woman should devote a lot of time to satisfying her husband."

Data show that almost all ethnic groups have a score of less than 2.5 for first statement. The rural Chinese in general have a slightly higher score than the rural Southern Thai Muslims, the Thais and the Thai Muslims respectively. However, among the urban respondents, the Thais have a slightly higher score than

TABLE 4.9

Attitudes toward Divorce and Remarriage by Ethnic Group

	Chinese				Thai			
	Rural		Urban		Rural		Urban	
Variable	Female	Male	Female	Male	Female	Male	Female	Male
Percentage Approving of a Woman Divorcing if								
They could not have children	28.7	42.1	30.5	39.0	42.1	50.9	36.2	36.3
He has a mistress	64.8	63.6	65.1	65.7	73.7	64.5	69.3	63.7
He is cruel to her	85.7	87.9	87.7	87.6	87.0	83.6	87.9	91.2
He does not support the family	84.7	92.5	90.6	87.6	90.4	85.5	91.6	94.1
She wants to marry another man	34.2	47.7	33.6	55.2	35.9	48.2	37.5	55.9
Percentage Approving of a Man Divorcing if								
They could not have children	39.1	29.0	38.4	29.5	53.6	43.6	47.4	30.4
She has a lover	89.3	89.7	91.2	94.3	94.1	93.6	92.9	96.1
She is cruel to him	81.8	79.5	85.6	85.7	83.3	79.1	83.6	86.3
She neglects the house and family	83.4	86.0	86.8	88.6	89.5	88.2	93.2	90.2
He wants to marry another woman	34.5	35.5	41.6	34.3	43.0	32.7	43.7	37.3

TABLE 4.9 (cont'd)

	Thai Muslim				Southern Thai Muslim			
	Rural		Urban		Rural		Urban	
Variable	Female	Male	Female	Male	Female	Male	Female	Male
Percentage Approving of a Woman Divorcing if								
They could not have children	39.1	56.3	33.3	41.4	32.0	33.7	19.2	28.1
He has a mistress	70.7	57.1	68.9	46.9	82.7	71.3	79.3	80.2
He is cruel to her	84.8	81.2	86.1	81.1	87.8	86.1	91.2	88.5
He does not support the family	92.3	87.5	86.8	83.8	86.3	84.1	91.7	88.5
She wants to marry another man	32.0	45.5	30.8	56.8	46.7	47.5	42.0	56.3
Percentage Approving of a Man Divorcing if								
They could not have children	54.2	42.0	41.2	32.4	31.0	30.7	23.8	31.2
She has a lover	90.6	92.9	89.0	91.0	85.8	88.1	88.6	90.6
She is cruel to him	80.5	86.6	83.3	76.6	83.8	86.1	88.1	93.8
She neglects the house and family	87.9	86.6	86.2	82.9	83.3	89.1	89.6	93.8
He wants to marry another woman	38.0	23.2	40.3	35.1	51.8	45.5	49.7	51.0

TABLE 4.9 (cont'd)
Attitudes toward Divorce and Remarriage by Ethnic Group

	Chinese				Thai			
	Rural		Urban		Rural		Urban	
Variable	Female	Male	Female	Male	Female	Male	Female	Male
Approval of a Widow Remarrying								
3 = Approve	57.0	71.1	53.7	62.9	68.1	83.6	67.8	75.5
2 = Depends on her age	12.7	8.4	18.9	17.1	14.6	6.4	11.8	7.8
1 = Disapprove	29.6	19.6	27.4	20.0	17.3	10.0	20.1	16.7
9 = Other	0.7	0.9	-	-	-	-	0.3	-
Total	100.0	100.0	100.0	100.0	100.0	100.0	100.0	100.0
Age after Which She Should No Longer Remarry	27.53	29.67	27.49	27.82	31.12	35.82	30.41	31.31
(Mean, Standard Deviation)	20.48	20.04	19.99	21.90	20.15	19.40	19.55	20.15

TABLE 4.9 (cont'd)

Variable	Thai Muslim				Southern Thai Muslim			
	Rural		Urban		Rural		Urban	
	Female	Male	Female	Male	Female	Male	Female	Male
Approval of a Widow Remarrying								
3 = Approve	73.4	75.9	67.3	76.6	61.4	77.2	60.6	68.8
2 = Depends on her age	8.8	8.0	11.9	12.6	12.2	5.9	11.9	12.4
1 = Disapprove	17.5	15.2	20.4	9.9	25.4	15.8	26.4	18.8
9 = Other	0.3	0.9	0.4	0.9	1.0	1.0	1.1	-
Total	100.0	100.0	100.0	100.0	100.0	100.0	100.0	100.0
Age after Which She Should No Longer Remarry	31.59	30.07	29.79	35.32	23.39	31.32	26.56	32.19
(Mean, Standard Deviation)	20.12	22.94	20.21	19.78	23.28	22.33	22.77	20.72

TABLE 4.10

Spouse Interaction and Sex Role Attitudes by Ethnic Group

Variable	Chinese				Thai			
	Rural		Urban		Rural		Urban	
	Female	Male	Female	Male	Female	Male	Female	Male
Ever Discussed Another Child								
2 = Yes	36.7	44.9	38.4	47.2	44.3	42.3	41.7	51.0
1 = No	63.3	55.1	61.6	52.8	55.7	57.7	58.3	49.0
Total	100.0	100.0	100.0	100.0	100.0	100.0	100.0	100.0
Shares Worries with Spouse								
4 = All the time	47.6	43.0	38.8	48.8	53.0	53.6	46.7	43.1
3 = Most of the time	19.9	18.7	23.8	27.9	22.4	22.7	25.1	27.5
2 = Sometimes	23.9	29.0	26.5	16.5	15.8	14.5	18.0	22.5
1 = Seldom	8.6	9.3	10.9	6.8	8.8	9.2	10.2	6.9
Total	100.0	100.0	100.0	100.0	100.0	100.0	100.0	100.0
Spouse Chosen to Spend Leisure Time with								
3 = First choice	81.3	66.8	78.6	79.1	80.5	69.5	84.3	72.8
2 = Alternate choice	18.7	33.2	21.4	20.9	19.5	30.5	15.3	25.9
1 = Not chosen	-	-	-	-	-	-	0.4	1.3
Total	100.0	100.0	100.0	100.0	100.0	100.0	100.0	100.0

TABLE 4.10 (cont'd)

Variable	Thai Muslim				Southern Thai Muslim			
	Rural		Urban		Rural		Urban	
	Female	Male	Female	Male	Female	Male	Female	Male
Ever Discussed Another Child								
2 = Yes	43.9	42.0	42.6	47.2	40.3	41.1	27.7	30.7
1 = No	56.1	58.0	57.4	52.8	59.7	58.9	72.3	69.3
Total	100.0	100.0	100.0	100.0	100.0	100.0	100.0	100.0
Shares Worries with Spouse								
4 = All the time	51.5	51.8	44.4	52.3	41.0	53.5	34.2	37.5
3 = Most of the time	20.9	21.4	22.3	16.2	32.0	28.7	30.6	30.2
2 = Sometimes	18.8	19.6	21.4	23.4	23.4	15.8	29.0	28.1
1 = Seldom	8.8	7.2	11.9	8.1	3.6	2.0	6.2	4.2
Total	100.0	100.0	100.0	100.0	100.0	100.0	100.0	100.0
Spouse Chosen to Spend Leisure Time with								
3 = First choice	68.7	59.8	43.6	36.0	79.5	69.3	77.9	68.2
2 = Alternate choice	31.3	40.2	56.1	63.1	20.0	30.7	22.1	31.8
1 = Not chosen	-	-	0.3	0.9	0.5	-	-	-
Total	100.0	100.0	100.0	100.0	100.0	100.0	100.0	100.0

TABLE 4.10 (cont'd)

Spouse Interaction and Sex Role Attitudes by Ethnic Group

Variable	Chinese				Thai			
	Rural		Urban		Rural		Urban	
	Female	Male	Female	Male	Female	Male	Female	Male
Mean Agreement With								
A girl becomes fully a woman only when she bears her own children	2.13	2.36	2.26	2.35	2.04	2.84	2.28	2.57
(Mean, Standard Deviation)	1.10	1.09	1.11	1.11	1.07	1.19	1.21	1.19
A Woman Should Devote A Lot of Time to Satisfying Her Husband	2.13	2.08	2.24	2.30	1.87	2.11	2.08	2.37
(Mean, Standard Deviation)	1.02	1.07	1.03	1.14	0.91	1.06	1.11	1.24
Wife Working Outside Home After Marriage								
3 = Good idea	63.5	52.3	67.0	62.9	66.4	64.5	73.7	65.7
2 = Indifferent	9.8	11.2	10.0	17.1	7.5	6.4	5.9	7.8
1 = Bad idea	26.7	36.5	23.0	20.0	26.1	29.1	20.4	26.5
Total	100.0	100.0	100.0	100.0	100.0	100.0	100.0	100.0
Wife Working If Husband's Earnings are Adequate								
2 = Approve	66.9	63.1	60.2	56.2	71.5	69.1	72.6	55.9
1 = Disapprove	33.1	36.9	39.8	43.8	28.5	30.9	27.4	44.1
Total	100.0	100.0	100.0	100.0	100.0	100.0	100.0	100.0

TABLE 4.10 (cont'd)

Variable	Thai Muslim				Southern Thai Muslim			
	Rural		Urban		Rural		Urban	
	Female	Male	Female	Male	Female	Male	Female	Male
Mean Agreement With								
A girl becomes fully a woman only when she bears her own children	1.95	2.47	2.17	2.40	2.10	2.15	2.08	2.16
(Mean, Standard Deviation)	1.05	1.16	1.19	1.27	0.98	1.02	0.86	0.89
A Woman Should Devote A Lot of Time to Satisfying Her Husband	1.80	1.96	1.90	1.95	1.66	1.61	1.89	1.70
(Mean, Standard Deviation)	0.92	0.97	1.04	1.07	0.74	0.87	0.80	0.78
Wife Working Outside Home After Marriage								
3 = Good idea	48.9	54.5	67.0	55.0	47.7	44.6	57.0	49.0
2 = Indifferent	8.9	4.5	6.3	8.1	5.6	6.9	6.7	11.5
1 = Bad idea	42.2	41.0	26.7	36.9	46.7	48.5	36.3	39.5
Total	100.0	100.0	100.0	100.0	100.0	100.0	100.0	100.0
Wife Working if Husband's Earnings are Adequate								
2 = Approve	52.1	44.6	45.7	41.4	92.2	89.1	83.1	80.2
1 = Disapprove	47.9	55.4	54.3	58.6	7.8	10.9	16.9	19.8
Total	100.0	100.0	100.0	100.0	100.0	100.0	100.0	100.0

the Chinese, the Thai Muslims and the Southern Thai Muslims, respectively. This suggests that agreement with the statement is relatively weak or at best neutral. Agreement to the statement that a women should devote a lot of time to satisfying her husband is even weaker than the first. The Chinese again have a higher agreement score than other ethnic groups, followed by the Thais, the Thai Muslims and the Southern Thai Muslims. Surprisingly the urban males and females show higher agreement scores than the rural respondents. This suggests that most respondents do not perceive women only as mothers and wives.

On the idea of the wife working outside the home after marriage, the Thais are most receptive to the idea, followed by the Chinese, the Thai Muslims and the Southern Thai Muslims. Less than half of the rural Thai Muslim and the Southern Thai Muslim women agreed with the idea. However, the data also show that the majority of the respondents, except the rural and urban Thai Muslim men and the urban Thai Muslim women, approve of the idea of the wife working even if husband's earnings are adequate.

In summary, the four ethnic groups differ a great deal not only in their fertility behaviour, but also in cultural and social orientations, ways of life, norms and values, and perceptions and attitudes towards values of children, divorce, remarriage, womanhood and role of women. It is, therefore, expected that the level of their fertility is affected differently by different sets of variables. In the next chapter, attempts will be made to analyse factors affecting the fertility behaviour of the four ethnic groups.

V

ANALYSIS OF THE RELATIONSHIP BETWEEN ETHNICITY AND FERTILITY

The present chapter will present a detailed analysis of the relationship between ethnicity and fertility. It will begin with analysis of variance and multiple classification analysis of the total number of children ever born to a woman (cumulative fertility), followed by an analysis of recent fertility (number of children born in the last five years) and the use of effective contraception, first with the total sample and then by ethnic group.

The use of MCA provides us with descriptive statistics in terms of proportion or mean differences as well as analytical statistics showing the relationships between dependent and independent variables first without control for any variables and then with control for the other independent variables and covariates. However, due to the fact that the available statistical package, SPSS, allows for only 5 independent variables and 5 covariates at a time it becomes cumbersome when one has more than 5 independent variables. Thus, instead of one model, many models of analysis have to be used by substituting one set of independent variables with another. This makes it somewhat difficult to evaluate the relative weight or significance of an independent variable in relation to the rest of variables that are used in the analysis. Furthermore, the number of cases of a particular category of a variable may change due to lack of information (missing values) of the variable or other variables involved in the analysis, making the mean value of a dependent variable change from table to table. However, if one is interested only in the pattern of differences, not in the absolute number, the problem can be disregarded.

In addition, an attempt is made to use multiple regression analysis, which includes all variables in the equation. To take care of the problematic disproportionate sample, multiple regression analysis is done by ethnic group. The effect of being a member of an ethnic group can be assessed by substituting the means of the variables of other ethnic group(s) in the regression equation of the group with which one wishes to compare and estimate the value(s) of the interested dependent variable(s).

Furthermore, three models of path analysis will be analysed: one dealing with the cumulative number of children ever born, another with recent fertility, and the last with the use of effective method of contraception. The use of path analysis is merely an attempt to order the variables in a theoretically casual manner. It should be noted that given the same set of variables, a different researcher with a different theoretical framework may order them differently. However, the ordering of the variables in the analysis is done collectively by the leaders of the research teams of the countries participating in the research project.

With the analysis of variance and the multiple classification analysis, it should be noted that only one model of analysis will be used with the total number of cases. For the model, ethnic group is treated as an independent variable. When analysis is done by ethnic group, ehtnicity is by definition left out of the analysis and other ethnic characteristics of variables are included in place.

ANOVA and MCA: Total Sample

The following analyses of variance of cumulative fertility, recent fertility and use of effective contraception involve the same set of independent variables and covariates. The model of analysis is specified as follows:

Specification of model(s)

Dependent Variable

CEB = Total number of children ever born

RF = Recent fertility

UEM = Use of effective method

Independent Variable

EG = Ethnic group

EAFF = Ethnic affiliation

EFERA = Ethnic fertility approval

HED = Husband's education

HOC = Husband's occupation

Covariates

CINC = Couple's income

PWR = Perceived woman's role

RELI = Religiosity

SPIN = Spouse interaction

MBF = Months of breastfeeding

<u>Number of Children Ever Born</u>

Insofar as the number of children ever born is concerned, the differences among the four ethnic groups are large enough to be statistically significant: The Thais average the lowest fertility, followed by the Chinese, the Southern Thai Muslims and the Thai Muslims (Tables 5.1 and 5.2). However, the degree of ethnic affiliation does not have any significant relationship with the dependent variable, but ethnic fertility approval is strongly and positively related to the fertility measure. The level of husband's education is significantly and negatively related to the dependent variable. Data also show that wives with husbands engaged in professional occupations have lowest fertility, followed by those who are engaged in services, farm and unclassified occupations respectively.

It is significant to note that the overall two-way interaction effects of the independent variables on the dependent variables are statistically significant. While the two independent variables -- husband's occupation and ethnic affiliation -- by themselves are not significant; their interaction is, however, significantly related to the dependent variable.

All the covariates are positively related to the dependent variable. Those who have higher incomes adhere to traditional roles of women, are more religious, have husbands who are more dominant in spouse relationship, breastfeed longer and average more live births than those who possess the opposite characteristics.

TABLE 5.1

ANOVA of Number of Children Ever Born (Total Sample)

Source of Variation	Sum of Squares	Degrees of Freedom	Mean Square	F Statistic	Significance of F
Main Effects	1,130.16	12	110.84	26.73	0.00
Ethnic group (V3)	97.43	3	32.47	7.83	0.00
Ethnic affiliation (V178)	7.99	2	3.99	0.96	0.38
Ethnic fertility approval (V179)	104.22	2	52.11	12.56	0.00
Husband's education (V53)	760.36	2	380.18	91.69	0.00
Husband's occupation (V75)	27.02	3	9.00	2.17	0.08
Covariates	406.22	5	81.24	19.59	0.00
Grouped couple's income	56.48	1	56.48	13.62	0.00
Perceived women's role	18.52	1	18.52	4.46	0.03
Religiosity	43.48	1	43.48	10.48	0.00
Spouse interaction	15.27	1	15.27	3.68	0.05
Months of breastfeeding	280.33	1	280.33	67.61	0.00

(cont'd on next page)

TABLE 5.1 (cont'd)

ANOVA of Number of Children Ever Born (Total Sample)

Source of Variation	Sum of Squares	Degrees of Freedom	Mean Square	F Statistic	Significance of F
2-Way Interactions	481.00	57	8.43	2.03	0.00
V3 x V178	11.74	6	1.95	0.47	0.83
V3 x V179	38.45	6	6.40	1.54	0.15
V3 x V53	67.71	6	11.28	2.72	0.01
V3 x V75	137.17	9	15.24	3.67	0.00
V178 x V179	5.37	4	1.34	0.32	0.86
V178 x V53	12.82	4	3.20	0.77	0.54
V178 x V75	92.43	6	15.40	3.71	0.00
V179 x V53	13.75	4	3.43	0.82	0.50
V179 x V75	55.86	6	9.31	2.24	0.03
V53 x V75	33.01	6	5.50	1.32	0.24
Explained	2,217.40	74	29.96	7.22	0.00
Residual	11,178.42	2,696	4.14		
Total	13,395.82	2,770			

Covariate	Raw Regression Coefficient
V183	0.08
V184	0.14
V185	0.04
V192	0.07
V195	0.20

TABLE 5.2

MCA of Number of Children Ever Born (Total Sample)
(Grand Mean = 3.00)

Variable & Category	N	Unadjusted Deviation	Adjusted Deviation
Ethnic Group			
Chinese	778	-0.09	0.06
Thai	829	-0.37	-0.20
Thai Muslim	607	0.36	0.18
Southern Thai Muslim	557	0.28	0.03
		(0.13)*	(0.06)**
Ethnic Affiliation			
Low	802	0.06	0.01
Medium	967	-0.12	-0.07
High	1,002	0.07	0.06
		(0.04)	(0.03)
Ethnic Fertility Approval			
Scores 1-3	35	-0.37	-0.44
Scores 4-6	1,600	-0.22	-0.15
Scores 7-9	1,136	0.23	0.23
		(0.12)	(0.09)
Husband's Education			
No schooling or primary	1,680	0.45	0.38
Some secondary	797	-0.45	-0.35
Post secondary	294	-1.35	-0.21
		(0.28)	(0.24)
Husband's Occupation			
Professional	1,447	-0.23	-0.05
Services, production	881	0.10	-0.00
Farm	346	0.58	0.15
Not classified	97	0.43	0.30
		(0.13)	(0.04)
Multiple R Squared		0.099	0.130
Multiple R		0.315	0.360

NOTES: In parentheses are Eta and Beta coefficients.

Recent Fertility

Regarding ethnic differentials in recent fertility, the data also show that the main effects of only two independent variables (ethnic group and husband's occupation) on recent fertility are statistically significant. The Thais average the lowest number of live births during the last 5 years, followed by the Chinese, the Southern Thai Muslims and the Thai Muslims (Tables 5.3 and 5.4). The other independent variables by themselves are not significantly related to recent fertility, but their two-way interactions are. Among the significant two-way interactions are ethnic group and ethnic fertility approval, ethnic group and husband occupation, ethnic affiliation and husband's education, and ethnic fertility approval and husband's occupation. The significant two-way interactions imply the significance of the ethnic variables to fertility.

Among the covariates, only two variables are significantly related to recent fertility. Duration of breastfeeding is found to be positively related to recent fertility, probably due to the fact that those who breastfeed longer were also from the lower socio-economic groups. Religiosity is found to be negatively related to recent fertility. This result is unexpected and could be due to the role of the recent religious movement in the sphere of birth control and social and economic development. The issue is another area of fruitful research.

Use of Effective Method

Most encouraging is the finding that all independent variables are significantly related to the use of effective methods of birth control. Only one covariate, spouse interaction, is found to be statistically significant (Tables 5.5 and 5.6). Data show that more Thais and the Chinese use more effective methods of contraception than the Thai Muslims. The Southern Thai Muslims use the least effective methods. Those who have strong ethnic affiliation are less likely to use effective methods than those who have lower ethnic affiliation. Furthermore, those who score low on ethnic fertility approval use more effective methods than those who score high. Data also show a strong linear correlation between education and use of effective contraceptive methods. It is also found that the farm families use less effective methods of birth control than those of the other occupational groups. Since the farmers are the majority of the country's population, there is more room for improving family planning programmes in the rural areas of the country.

TABLE 5.3

ANOVA of Recent Fertility (Total Sample)

Source of Variation	Sum of Squares	Degrees of Freedom	Mean Square	F Statistic	Significance of F
Main Effects	43.89	12	3.65	4.54	0.00
Ethnic group (V3)	26.92	3	8.97	11.14	0.00
Ethnic affiliation (V178)	0.83	2	0.41	0.51	0.59
Ethnic fertility approval (V179)	2.62	2	1.31	1.62	0.19
Husband's education (V53)	2.92	2	1.46	1.81	0.16
Husband's occupation (V75)	13.79	3	4.59	5.70	0.00
Covariates	179.32	5	35.86	44.52	0.00
Grouped couple's income	1.04	1	1.04	1.29	0.25
Perceived women's role	0.00	1	0.00	0.01	0.91
Religiosity	15.85	1	15.85	19.68	0.00
Spouse interaction	0.02	1	0.02	0.02	0.86
Months of breastfeeding	163.78	1	163.78	203.31	0.00

(cont'd on next page)

TABLE 5.3 (cont'd)

ANOVA of Recent Fertility (Total Sample)

Source of Variation	Sum of Squares	Degrees of Freedom	Mean Square	F Statistic	Significance of F
2-Way Interactions	65.72	57	1.15	1.43	0.01
V3 x V178	4.22	6	0.70	0.87	0.51
V3 x V179	11.49	6	1.91	2.37	0.02
V3 x V53	2.79	6	0.46	0.57	0.74
V3 x V75	13.85	9	1.54	1.91	0.04
V178 x V179	2.06	4	0.51	0 64	0.63
V178 x V53	8.32	4	2.08	2.58	0.03
V178 x V75	1.26	6	0.21	0.26	0.95
V179 x V53	0.99	4	0.24	0.30	0.87
V179 x V75	15.98	6	2.66	3.30	0.00
V53 x V75	2.04	6	0.34	0.42	0.86
Explained	288.94	74	3.90	4.84	0.00
Residual	2,171.72	2,696	0.80		
Total	2,460.67	2,770	0.88		

Covariate	Raw Regression Coefficient
V183	-0.01
V184	-0.00
V185	-0.25
V192	-0.00
V195	-0.15

TABLE 5.4
MCA of Recent Fertility (Total Sample)
(Grand Mean = 0.76)

Variable & Category	N	Unadjusted Deviation	Adjusted Deviation
Ethnic Group			
Chinese	778	0.03	0.02
Thai	829	-0.10	-0.15
Thai Muslim	607	0.14	0.14
Southern Thai Muslim	557	-0.06	0.04
		(0.10)	(0.11)
Ethnic Affiliation			
Low	802	0.02	-0.02
Medium	967	0.01	0.03
High	1,002	-0.02	-0.01
		(0.02)	(0.02)
Ethnic Fertility Approval			
Scores 1-3	35	-0.16	-0.18
Scores 4-6	1,600	-0.02	-0.01
Scores 7-9	1,136	0.04	0.02
		(0.04)	(0.03)
Husband's Education			
No schooling or primary	1,680	0.00	-0.04
Some secondary	797	0.03	0.07
Post secondary	294	-0.09	0.05
		(0.04)	(0.06)
Husband's Occupation			
Professional	1,447	-0.05	-0.04
Services, production	881	0.07	0.06
Farm	346	0.04	0.01
Not classified	97	-0.01	-0.01
		(0.06)	(0.05)
Multiple R Squared		0.018	0.091
Multiple R		0.134	0.301

NOTES: In parentheses are Eta and Beta coefficients.

TABLE 5.5

ANOVA of Use of Effective Contraception: Model (Total Sample)

Source of Variation	Sum of Squares	Degrees of Freedom	Mean Square	F Statistic	Significance of F
Main Effects	446.87	12	37.24	50.10	0.00
Ethnic group (V3)	314.45	3	104.81	141.03	0.00
Ethnic affiliation (V178)	5.12	2	2.56	3.44	0.03
Ethnic fertility approval (V179)	6.19	2	3.09	4.16	0.01
Husband's education (V53)	11.65	2	5.82	7.84	0.00
Husband's occupation (V75)	12.88	3	4.29	5.78	0.00
Covariates	9.52	5	1.90	2.56	0.02
Grouped couple's income	1.65	1	1.65	2.22	0.13
Perceived women's role	0.39	1	0.39	0.52	0.46
Religiosity	1.38	1	1.38	1.86	0.17
Spouse interaction	3.78	1	3.78	5.09	0.02
Months of breastfeeding	2.23	1	2.23	3.01	0.08

(cont'd on next page)

TABLE 5.5 (cont'd)

ANOVA of Use of Effective Contraception: Model (Total Sample)

Source of Variation	Sum of Squares	Degrees of Freedom	Mean Square	F Statistic	Significance of F
2-Way Interactions	48.76	56	0.87	1.17	0.18
V3 x V178	8.71	6	1.45	1.95	0.06
V3 x V179	1.95	6	0.32	0.43	0.85
V3 x V53	3.97	6	0.66	0.89	0.50
V3 x V75	7.35	9	0.81	1.10	0.35
V178 x V179	4.76	4	1.19	1.60	0.17
V178 x V53	3.01	4	0.75	1.01	0.39
V178 x V75	2.15	6	0.35	0.48	0.82
V179 x V53	0.11	3	0.03	0.05	0.98
V179 x V75	3.22	6	0.53	0.72	0.63
V53 x V75	5.93	6	0.98	1.33	0.24
Explained	505.16	73	6.92	9.31	0.00
Residual	1,944.97	2,617	0.74		
Total	2,450.13	2,690	0.91		

Covariate	Raw Regression Coefficient
V183	0.01
V184	-0.02
V185	-0.00
V192	-0.03
V195	0.01

TABLE 5.6
MCA of Use of Effective Contraception (Total Sample)
(Grand Mean = 1.27)

Variable & Category	N	Unadjusted Deviation	Adjusted Deviation
Ethnic Group			
Chinese	754	0.26	0.19
Thai	793	0.26	0.25
Thai Muslim	599	0.00	0.02
Southern Thai Muslim	545	-0.74	-0.64
		(0.40)	(0.35)
Ethnic Affiliation			
Low	791	0.01	0.02
Medium	932	0.09	0.05
High	968	-0.09	-0.06
		(0.08)	(0.05)
Ethnic Fertility Approval			
Scores 1-3	34	0.29	0.23
Scores 4-6	1550	0.09	0.03
Scores 7-9	1170	-0.14	-0.05
		(0.12)	(0.05)
Husband's Education			
No schooling or primary	1643	-0.10	-0.06
Some secondary	760	0.18	0.09
Post secondary	288	0.12	0.11
		(0.14)	(0.08)
Husband's Occupation			
Professional	1395	0.11	0.02
Services, production	862	-0.01	0.03
Farm	340	-0.40	-0.19
Not classified	94	0.01	0.06
		(0.17)	(0.07)
Multiple R Squared		0.182	0.186
Multiple R		0.427	0.432

NOTES: In parentheses are Eta and Beta coefficients.

ANOVA and MCA by Ethnic Group

Due to the fact that the sample drawn was based on a quota number of each ethnic group to be sampled, the proportional distribution of the sample by ethnic group is not the same as the proportional distribution of the population. Even if the sample of each ethnic group is be representative of its own ethnic population, it is most inappropriate to analyse the effects of all the independent variables by treating all cases as one sample as they are not properly weighted according to their proportions in the national population. An appropriate way to cope with the problem is to analyse the data by ethnic group.

There are 5 models of analysis for each dependent variable. All models share the same set of covariates. The models are specified as follows:

Specification of Model(s)

	Model I	Model II	Model III	Model IV	Model V
Dependent					
	CEB	CEB	CEB	CEB	CEB
	RF	RF	RF	RF	RF
	UEM	UEM	UEM	UEM	UEM
Independent					
	EAFF	EAFF	EAFF	EAFF	EAFF
	EFERA	EFERA	EFERA	EFERA	EFERA
	HED	FEM	HTYPE	ACCONT	DFS
	HOC	GENB	HDOM	DFS	FECUM
	WED	SONPRE	PSYCOS	FECUN	CMOR
Covariates					
	CINC	CINC	CINC	CINC	CINC
	PWR	PWR	PWR	PWR	PWR
	RELI	RELI	RELI	RELI	RELI
	SPIN	SPIN	SPIN	SPIN	SPIN
	MBF	MBF	MBF	MBF	MBF

Further Specifications of the Variable

As some variables have already been specified, the rest are specified as follows:

WED = Wife's education

FEM = Female employment

GENB = Gender balance of children

SONPRE = Son preference

HTYPE = Household type

HDOM = Husband's dominance

PSYCOS = Psychic cost of contraception

ACCONT = Access to contraceptive service

DFS = Desired family size

FECUN = Perceived fecundity

CMOR = Child mortality experience

When the same models of analysis are used, the behaviour of each independent variable in different ethnic groups is more readily observable than otherwise. The presentation of the analysis will begin with the analysis of cumulative fertility or total number of children ever born, followed by recent fertility, and then the use of effective methods of birth control.

Since the effects of ethnic affiliation (EAFF) and ethnic fertility approval (EFERA) are presented in Model I, they will not be shown again in other Models which include them as the independent variables. This means that MCA tables showing the results of analysis based on Models II to V will be truncated by omitting the patterns of the relationship of the dependent variable(s) and the two variables (EFERA and EAFF).

Fertility Measures by Age and Ethnic Group

Before the results of analysis of variance and multiple classification analysis of factors affecting the dependent variable(s) are presented, a set of tables which cross-tabulate the dependent variable(s) by ethnic group and age group will provide a brief overview of ethnic differences in cumulative fertility, recent fertility and use of effective method(s).

Table 5.7 shows the averaged number of children ever born by age group and ethnicity. The data clearly show that the number of children ever born increases with the age of women. The Thais average lowest number of children ever born (2.44 for the urban, 2.80 for the rural), followed by the Chinese, the Southern Thai Muslims and the Thai Muslims. The last ethnic group average 3.56 children in the rural areas and 2.94 in the urban areas.

What is more important is the fact that those who have high cumulative fertility also have high recent fertility. Table 5.8 shows that the Thais have lowest recent fertility while the Thai Muslims have highest recent fertility. In addition, the data also show that their actual cumulative and recent fertility match their desired family size. Those who have higher fertility also desire a larger family size (Table 5.9). The average desired family size of the urban and rural Thais are 2.97 and 3.19 compared with 3.42 and 3.53 of the Chinese, and 3.66 and 4.03 of the Thai Muslims and 3.93 and 4.21 of the Southern Thai Muslims in the urban and rural areas, respectively.

Consistently, the percentage practising effective family planning is greatest among the Thais, closely followed by the Chinese, the Thai Muslims and the Southern Thai Muslims. Slightly over one-third of the Southern Thai Muslims currently practise family planning compared with three-fifths of the Thais and the Chinese (Table 5.10). Even though only one-third of the Southern Thai Muslims reported that they are practising contraception, it is considered a major improvement. In the past very few admitted they ever practised it. It is suspected that the Muslims' contraceptive use rate is much higher than is reported. Under-reporting may be the result of certain religious sanctions against birth control.

Total Number of Children Ever Born

Model I

According to Model I, the analysis of variance shows that ethnic affiliation is not significantly related to the cumulative fertility for all ethnic groups (Tables 5.11 and 5.12). This is probably due to the fact that over a lifetime there are many other factors that are more significant to childbearing than just ethnic affiliation.

Among the Chinese, data show that husband's occupation, husband's education and wife's education are significantly related to the number of children ever born. As for the Thais, it has been found that education of both wife and husband is significantly and negatively related to fertility while husband's occupation is not. More significant and policy relevant is the finding that ethnic fertility approval is positively related to the dependent variable. Obviously, this suggests that planners should be aware of and sensitive to the existence of such ethnic attitudes. Similar to the Thais, the Thai Muslims and the Southern Thai Muslims also show that education of husband and wife and ethnic fertility approval are significantly related to the number of children ever born.

It should be noted that while husband's occupation is not significantly related to the number of children ever born among the Thais, the Thai Muslims, and the Southern Thai Muslims, it is a significant variable for the Chinese. The finding implies that among the Chinese, some occupations encourage higher fertility than others. However, education of both husband and wife also significantly affects their fertility behaviour.

Model II

In Model II, three independent variables -- HED, WED and HOC -- are replaced by FEM, GENB and SONPRE, and the other two independent variables are ethnic affiliation and ethnic fertility approval. These two variables are kept in all models of analysis to be presented. The focus of this model is on the behaviour of female employment (FEM), gender balance of living children (GENB) and son preference (SONPRE).

Analysis of the data shows that gender balance of living children is significantly related to the total number of children ever born among the Chinese, the Thais and the Thai Muslims but not among the Southern Thai Muslims (Tables 5.13 and 5.14). This is probably due to the fact that the Chinese and the Thai Muslims have a strong preference for sons, and the Thais attempt to have children of both sexes. It has been found that the Thais in general express a more moderate preference for sons than the Chinese do. Female employment is found to be significant only among the Southern Thai Muslims. It is interesting to note that among the Southern Thai Muslim women, those who work far away from home average more live births than those who work at home or those who do not work. The finding implies that the Southern

TABLE 5.7

The Mean Number of Children Ever Born by Ethnicity and Age-Group

	Chinese				Thai			
	Rural		Urban		Rural		Urban	
Wife's Age	N	Mean	N	Mean	N	Mean	N	Mean
15 - 19	-	-	2	0.0	7	0.28	3	1.33
20 - 24	35	0.9	28	0.82	65	1.28	72	1.21
25 - 29	98	2.18	103	2.01	114	1.90	106	1.86
30 - 34	101	2.74	121	2.58	79	2.77	107	2.50
35 - 39	81	3.74	97	3.48	89	3.49	65	3.37
40 - 44	80	4.15	64	4.22	62	4.52	62	3.42
45 - 49	19	4.79	7	5.71	17	5.88	9	5.22
Total	414	3.02	422	2.82	433	2.80	424	2.44

TABLE 5.7 (cont'd)

	Thai Muslim				Southern Thai Muslim			
	Rural		Urban		Rural		Urban	
Wife's Age	N	Mean	N	Mean	N	Mean	N	Mean
15 - 19	16	0.25	8	0.38	20	0.55	20	0.70
20 - 24	67	1.37	69	1.38	67	1.28	61	1.74
25 - 29	110	2.62	124	1.93	60	2.32	64	2.30
30 - 34	71	3.92	91	2.96	53	3.68	60	3.57
35 - 39	76	4.53	57	4.39	40	4.90	31	5.71
40 - 44	61	6.31	68	5.07	50	5.44	38	5.45
45 - 49	8	8.00	12	4.92	7	6.86	14	7.21
Total	409	3.56	429	2.94	297	3.14	289	3.36

TABLE 5.8

The Mean Number of Children Ever Born During the Past Five Years by Ethnicity and Age-Group

	Chinese				Thai			
	Rural		Urban		Rural		Urban	
Wife's Age	N	Mean	N	Mean	N	Mean	N	Mean
15 - 19	-	-	2	0.00	7	0.28	3	1.33
20 - 24	35	0.77	28	0.57	65	0.85	72	0.86
25 - 29	98	1.17	103	1.19	114	1.01	106	0.92
30 - 34	101	1.08	121	1.00	79	0.72	107	0.64
35 - 39	81	0.62	97	0.63	89	0.44	65	0.45
40 - 44	80	0.31	64	0.28	62	0.29	62	0.16
45 - 49	19	0.16	7	0.14	17	0.35	9	0.00
Total	414	0.79	422	0.81	433	0.67	424	0.64

TABLE 5.8 (cont'd)

	Thai Muslim				Southern Thai Muslim			
	Rural		Urban		Rural		Urban	
Wife's Age	N	Mean	N	Mean	N	Mean	N	Mean
15 - 19	16	0.12	8	0.38	20	0.35	20	0.50
20 - 24	67	0.82	69	0.94	67	0.70	61	1.00
25 - 29	110	1.24	124	0.90	60	0.80	64	0.94
30 - 34	71	0.96	91	0.80	53	0.77	60	0.83
35 - 39	76	0.67	57	0.47	40	0.42	31	0.71
40 - 44	61	0.48	68	0.31	50	0.36	38	0.47
45 - 49	8	0.50	12	0.08	7	0.28	14	0.36
Total	409	0.84	429	0.70	297	0.61	289	0.78

TABLE 5.9
Average Desired Family Size by Ethnicity and Age-Group

	Chinese				Thai			
	Rural		Urban		Rural		Urban	
Wife's Age	N	Mean	N	Mean	N	Mean	N	Mean
15 - 19	-	-	2	3.00	7	2.28	3	1.67
20 - 24	35	2.77	28	2.32	65	2.52	72	2.38
25 - 29	98	2.94	103	2.98	114	2.57	106	2.58
30 - 34	101	3.37	121	3.16	79	3.23	107	3.01
35 - 39	81	3.90	97	3.81	89	3.66	65	3.60
40 - 44	80	4.12	64	4.33	62	4.13	62	3.42
45 - 49	19	4.84	7	5.00	17	4.29	9	4.78
Total	414	3.53	422	3.42	433	3.19	424	2.97

TABLE 5.9 (cont'd)

Wife's Age	Thai Muslim				Southern Thai Muslim			
	Rural		Urban		Rural		Urban	
	N	Mean	N	Mean	N	Mean	N	Mean
15 - 19	16	2.06	8	2.00	20	2.80	20	3.10
20 - 24	67	2.84	69	3.07	67	3.31	61	3.02
25 - 29	110	3.75	124	3.05	60	4.15	64	3.52
30 - 34	71	4.25	91	4.01	53	4.58	60	3.90
35 - 39	76	4.45	57	4.24	40	5.05	31	5.42
40 - 44	61	5.43	68	3.38	50	4.90	38	4.89
45 - 49	8	5.38	12	4.83	7	4.71	14	5.21
Total	409	4.03	429	3.66	297	4.21	289	3.93

TABLE 5.10

Proportion (p) of Women Using Effective Contraception by Ethnicity and Age

	Chinese				Thai			
	Rural		Urban		Rural		Urban	
Wife's Age	N	Mean	N	Mean	N	Mean	N	Mean
15 - 19	-	-	2	0.78	7	0.33	3	0.00
20 - 24	31	0.53	28	0.62	65	0.56	69	0.46
25 - 29	94	0.60	102	0.58	114	0.61	101	0.69
30 - 34	94	0.59	121	0.59	72	0.61	100	0.70
35 - 39	80	0.61	97	0.65	87	0.61	62	0.61
40 - 44	75	0.59	63	0.55	60	0.54	54	0.58
45 - 49	16	0.39	7	0.55	17	0.59	9	0.47
Total	390		420		422		398	

TABLE 5.10 (cont'd)

Wife's Age	Thai Muslim				Southern Thai Muslim			
	Rural		Urban		Rural		Urban	
	N	Mean	N	Mean	N	Mean	N	Mean
15 - 19	16	0.30	8	0.19	20	0.34	20	0.29
20 - 24	67	0.40	65	0.51	67	0.37	57	0.32
25 - 29	110	0.46	122	0.58	59	0.33	63	0.39
30 - 34	70	0.57	89	0.57	52	0.37	60	0.37
35 - 39	75	0.52	57	0.53	40	0.31	31	0.34
40 - 44	58	0.43	68	0.51	49	0.35	34	0.36
45 - 49	8	0.19	12	0.45	7	0.00	14	0.28
Total	404		421		294		280	

TABLE 5.11

ANOVA of Live Birth: Model I

Source of Variation	Significance of F				
	Total	Chinese	Thai	Thai Muslim	Southern Thai Muslim
Main Effects	0.000	0.000	0.000	0.000	0.000
Ethnic affiliation (V178)	0.084	0.639	0.339	0.879	0.758
Ethnic fertility approval (V179)	0.000	0.310	0.006	0.003	0.004
Husband's education (V53)	0.000	0.000	0.000	0.003	0.007
Husband's occupation (V75)	0.099	0.001	0.293	0.310	0.057
Wife's education (V55)	0.000	0.000	0.001	0.000	0.000
Covariates	0.000	0.000	0.000	0.000	0.004
Couple's income	0.000	0.001	0.240	0.138	0.007
Perceived women's role	0.007	0.630	0.142	0.439	0.110
Religiosity	0.000	0.497	0.047	0.011	0.266
Spouse interaction	0.017	0.794	0.081	0.063	0.676
Months of breastfeeding	0.000	0.000	0.000	0.002	0.022

(cont'd on next page)

TABLE 5.11 (cont'd)

ANOVA of Live Birth: Model I

Source of Variation	Significance of F				
	Total	Chinese	Thai	Thai Muslim	Southern Thai Muslim
2-Way Interactions	0.040	0.439	0.778	0.242	0.123
V178 x V179	0.479	0.072	0.948	0.662	0.820
V178 x V53	0.806	0.596	0.679	0.512	0.964
V178 x V75	0.013	0.445	0.066	0.001	0.020
V178 x V55	0.059	0.763	0.745	0.588	0.746
V179 x V53	0.514	0.986	0.668	0.092	0.306
V179 x V75	0.026	0.023	0.728	0.654	0.406
V179 x V55	0.323	0.398	0.769	0.758	0.204
V53 x V75	0.301	0.568	0.119	0.346	0.072
V53 x V55	0.604	0.428	0.740	0.485	0.094
V75 x V55	0.896	0.735	0.120	0.543	0.349
Explained	0.000	0.000	0.000	0.000	0.000
Covariate Raw Regression Coefficient					
Couple's income	0.107	0.097	0.056	0.091	0.234
Perceived women's role	0.173	0.054	0.158	0.120	0.281
Religiosity	0.049	0.013	0.042	0.067	0.059
Spouse interaction	0.092	0.016	0.109	0.177	0.044
Months of breastfeeding	0.184	0.217	0.185	0.207	0.120

TABLE 5.12
MCA of Live Birth: Model I

Variable & Category	N	Total (Grand Mean = 3.00) Unadjusted Deviation	Adjusted Deviation
Ethnic Affiliation		(0.04)	(0.03)
Low	802	0.06	0.11
Medium	967	-0.12	-0.08
High	1002	0.07	-0.01
Ethnic Fertility Approval		(0.12)	(0.09)
Scores 1-3	35	-0.37	-0.54
Scores 4-6	1600	-0.22	-0.16
Scores 7-9	1136	0.32	0.24
Husband's Education		(0.28)	(0.16)
No schooling or primary	1680	0.45	0.25
Some secondary	797	-0.45	-0.25
Post secondary	294	-1.35	-0.76
Husband's Occupation		(0.13)	(0.04)
Professional	1447	-0.23	-0.04
Services production	881	0.10	-0.02
Farm	346	0.58	0.13
Not classified	97	0.43	0.29
Wife's Education		(0.29)	(0.19)
No schooling or primary	2069	0.36	0.24
Some secondary	556	-0.90	-0.61
Post secondary	146	-1.63	-0.04
Multiple R Squared		0.120	0.153
Multiple R		0.347	0.391

TABLE 5.12 (cont'd)

Chinese (Grand Mean = 2.91)			Thai (Grand Mean = 2.64)		
N	Unadjusted Deviation	Adjusted Deviation	N	Unadjusted Deviation	Adjusted Deviation
	(0.01)	(0.02)		(0.05)	(0.04)
369	0.01	0.03	11	0.46	-0.52
249	-0.03	-0.06	349	0.09	-0.06
160	0.01	0.01	469	0.08	0.05
	(0.06)	(0.05)		(0.11)	(0.10)
4	0.84	0.96	16	-1.20	-1.30
495	-0.08	-0.06	549	-0.06	-0.02
279	0.13	0.09	264	0.20	0.12
	(0.30)	(0.22)		(0.23)	(0.12)
429	0.43	0.32	451	0.28	0.12
267	-0.30	-0.24	282	-0.06	0.02
82	-1.25	-0.90	96	-1.13	-0.61
	(0.13)	(0.12)		(0.11)	(0.07)
586	0.01	0.05	357	-0.22	-0.06
141	-0.23	-0.25	346	0.14	0.07
33	1.03	0.70	99	0.14	-0.17
18	-0.52	-0.86	27	0.59	0.56
	(0.26)	(0.16)		(0.23)	(0.15)
560	0.29	0.18	612	0.24	0.16
187	-0.67	-0.42	160	-0.50	-0.34
31	-1.30	-0.74	57	-1.18	-0.73
	0.133	0.174		0.086	0.118
	0.364	0.417		0.294	0.343

TABLE 5.12 (cont'd)
MCA of Live Birth: Model I

Variable & Category	Thai Muslim (Grand Mean = 3.18)			Southern Thai Muslim (Grand Mean = 3.04)		
	N	Unadjusted Deviation	Adjusted Deviation	N	Unadjusted Deviation	Adjusted Deviation
Ethnic Affiliation		(0.05)	(0.02)		(0.11)	(0.05)
Low	274	-0.09	0.00	148	-0.19	0.19
Medium	204	-0.04	-0.06	165	-0.27	-0.03
High	129	0.26	0.09	244	0.30	-0.09
Ethnic Fertility Approval		(0.16)	(0.12)		(0.12)	(0.12)
Scores 1-3	11	0.18	0.11	4	0.47	0.01
Scores 4-6	317	-0.40	-0.30	239	-0.34	-0.36
Scores 7-9	279	0.45	0.33	314	0.25	0.27
Husband's Education		(0.26)	(0.15)		(0.33)	(0.14)
No schooling or primary	409	0.48	0.27	391	0.51	0.21
Some secondary	144	-0.87	-0.51	104	-0.87	-0.34
Post secondary	54	-1.29	-0.68	62	-1.77	-0.76
Husband's Occupation		(0.18)	(0.06)		(0.20)	(0.11)
Professional	299	-0.41	-0.15	205	-0.55	-0.07
Services production	188	0.27	0.12	206	0.15	-0.08
Farm	90	0.89	0.25	124	0.36	0.01
Not classified	30	-0.23	-0.07	22	1.67	1.35
Wife's Education		(0.27)	(0.16)		(0.41)	(0.33)
No schooling or primary	473	0.36	0.22	424	0.56	0.45
Some secondary	115	-1.15	-0.69	94	-1.64	-1.33
Post secondary	19	-2.10	-1.23	39	-2.15	-1.70
Multiple R Squared		0.123	0.155		0.209	0.234
Multiple R		0.350	0.393		0.457	0.483

NOTE: In parentheses are Eta and Beta coefficients.

TABLE 5.13
ANOVA of Live Birth: Model II

Source of Variation	Significance of F				
	Total	Chinese	Thai	Thai Muslim	Southern Thai Muslim
Main Effects	0.000	0.000	0.000	0.000	0.000
Ethnic affiliation (V178)	0.022	0.291	0.619	0.521	0.035
Ethnic fertility approval (V179)	0.000	0.367	0.058	0.033	0.001
Wife's education (V79)	0.194	0.762	0.459	0.776	0.009
Gender balance (V186)	0.000	0.000	0.000	0.000	0.000
Son preference (V187)	0.314	0.099	0.835	0.800	0.202
Covariates	0.000	0.055	0.003	0.501	0.337
Couple's income	0.746	0.019	0.062	0.831	0.531
Perceived women's role	0.001	0.182	0.102	0.099	0.195
Religiosity	0.001	0.770	0.191	0.820	0.609
Spouse interaction	0.912	0.477	0.275	0.683	0.796
Months of breastfeeding	0.000	0.088	0.002	0.256	0.087
2-Way Interactions	0.546	0.325	0.806	0.645	0.014
Explained	0.000	0.000	0.000	0.000	0.000
Covariate Raw Regression Coefficient					
Couple's income	0.009	0.080	-0.123	0.016	-0.073
Perceived women's role	0.229	-0.166	0.197	0.291	0.250
Religiosity	0.038	0.007	0.030	0.007	0.029
Spouse interaction	0.005	-0.048	0.078	-0.045	-0.030
Months of breastfeeding	0.116	0.086	0.151	0.091	0.102

TABLE 5.14
MCA of Live Birth: Model II

Variable & Category	Chinese (Grand Mean = 2.75)			Thai (Grand Mean = 2.53)		
	N	Unadjusted Deviation	Adjusted Deviation	N	Unadjusted Deviation	Adjusted Deviation
Wife's Employment		(0.08)	(0.04)		(0.05)	(0.10)
Never worked	93	-0.17	0.15	163	-0.12	-0.28
Work at home	405	-0.01	-0.02	321	0.08	0.08
Work far away	20	-0.65	-0.21	81	-0.06	0.24
Gender Balance		(0.52)	(0.49)		(0.49)	(0.45)
No children	59	-2.64	-2.49	80	-2.31	-2.14
Balance	151	0.20	0.21	137	0.34	0.31
Imbalance	151	-0.20	0.21	137	0.34	0.31
Son Preference		(0.07)	(0.06)		(0.03)	(0.00)
More sons	440	0.06	0.05	402	0.04	0.00
More daughters	70	-0.32	-0.27	163	-0.09	-0.00
Multiple R Squared		0.281	0.297		0.246	0.271
Multiple R		0.531	0.545		0.496	0.520

TABLE 5.14 (cont'd)

Variable & Category	Thai Muslim (Grand Mean = 3.18)			Southern Thai Muslim (Grand Mean = 3.04)		
	N	Unadjusted Deviation	Adjusted Deviation	N	Unadjusted Deviation	Adjusted Deviation
Wife's Employment		(0.11)	(0.03)		(0.20)	(0.15)
Never worked	97	0.25	0.05	175	-0.51	-0.39
Work at home	254	0.07	0.03	151	0.55	0.35
Work far away	64	-0.67	-0.20	38	0.17	0.42
Gender Balance		(0.46)	(0.43)		(0.52)	(0.46)
No children	72	-2.57	-2.37	55	-0.95	-2.57
Balance	114	0.28	0.17	117	0.94	0.85
Imbalance	229	0.67	0.66	192	0.27	0.22
Son Preference		(0.04)	(0.02)		(0.08)	(0.06)
More sons	293	0.06	0.03	250	0.13	0.10
More daughters	122	-0.14	-0.07	114	-0.29	-0.22
Multiple R Squared		0.234	0.242		0.329	0.339
Multiple R		0.483	0.492		0.573	0.582

Thai Muslims work only when they have large families. In general the wives of the Southern Thai Muslims normally stay at home unless there are compelling economic reasons. It is also noteworthy that the two-way interactions of the independent variables are significant only for the Southern Thai Muslims, suggesting a stronger impact of the independent variable than that shown by the significance of the effects of the variables.

Further, multiple classification analysis of live births shows that for all ethnic groups, gender imbalance is positively related to higher fertility, suggesting that couples will attempt to achieve gender balance even if this means producing more children. The Southern Thai Muslims, more so than the Thai Muslims, the Chinese and the Thais respectively, exhibit higher fertility when there is gender imbalance. Further examination of son preference and level of fertility shows that the difference between those who prefer sons to daughters and those who prefer the opposite is the least among the Thais, and highest among the Southern Thai Muslims, followed in decreasing order by the Thai Muslims and the Chinese (Table 5.14).

Model III

In Model III, the focus is on the behaviour of HTYPE, HDOM and PSYCOS. Analysis of data shows that household type is a variable significantly related to cumulative fertility among the Chinese, the Thais and the Thai Muslims but not among the Southern Thai Muslims, and that husband's dominance is significant only among the Chinese. The two-way interactions of the variables are not statistically significant (Tables 5.15 and 5.16).

Multiple classification analysis further shows that those who live in a joint household with three couples or more average a lower number of live births than those who live in a joint household with two couples or less or in a nuclear household, respectively. The result is not expected but explainable. Space and economic constraints could been the reasons for such a phenomenon. As for the behaviour of husband's dominance, the data show that for all ethnic groups, egalitarian couples average lower fertility than non-egalitarian couples. Lower fertility is experienced in Chinese families where the wife's influence is dominant. This result is expected.

Model IV

Model IV of analysis focuses on the behavioural effects of

TABLE 5.15
ANOVA of Live Birth: Model III

Source of Variation	Significance of F				
	Total	Chinese	Thai	Thai Muslim	Southern Thai Muslim
Main Effects	0.000	0.007	0.000	0.000	0.029
Ethnic affiliation (V178)	0.096	0.937	0.450	0.426	0.052
Ethnic fertility approval (V179)	0.000	0.189	0.003	0.000	0.015
Household types (V49)	0.000	0.001	0.000	0.001	0.191
Wife influence (V193)	0.179	0.031	0.638	0.834	0.397
Psychic cost of contraception (V197)	0.374	0.838	0.272	0.034	0.840
Covariates	0.000	0.000	0.000	0.000	0.000
Couple's income	0.002	0.000	0.774	0.804	0.305
Perceived women's role	0.001	0.314	0.368	0.173	0.006
Religiosity	0.000	0.716	0.022	0.016	0.271
Spouse interaction	0.376	0.516	0.205	0.371	0.819
Months of breastfeeding	0.000	0.000	0.000	0.000	0.000
2-Way Interactions	0.608	0.084	0.436	0.881	0.086
Explained	0.000	0.000	0.000	0.000	0.000
Covariate Raw Regression Coefficient					
Couple's income	0.071	0.102	-0.013	0.015	0.095
Perceived women's role	0.226	-0.115	0.099	0.222	0.530
Religiosity	0.047	-0.007	0.049	0.066	0.064
Spouse interaction	0.035	-0.040	0.080	0.089	-0.026
Months of breastfeeding	0.284	0.293	0.260	0.318	0.229

TABLE 5.16
MCA of Live Birth: Model III

Variable & Category	Chinese (Grand Mean = 2.93)			Thai (Grand Mean = 2.64)		
	N	Unadjusted Deviation	Adjusted Deviation	N	Unadjusted Deviation	Adjusted Deviation
Household Types		(0.13)	(0.17)		(0.14)	(0.15)
Nuclear	501	0.18	0.25	561	0.16	0.18
Joint (one couple)	227	-0.28	-0.42	197	-0.17	-0.26
Joint (2 or more couples)	65	-0.37	-0.44	76	-0.73	-0.69
Wife Influence		(0.09)	(0.09)		(0.04)	(0.04)
Husband	351	0.15	0.15	338	0.04	0.03
Equal	126	-0.34	-0.31	52	0.11	0.11
Wife	316	-0.03	-0.04	344	-0.09	-0.08
Psychic Cost of Contraception		(0.03)	(0.03)		(0.05)	(0.07)
Low	227	-0.04	-0.02	210	0.12	0.17
Medium	352	-0.02	-0.05	342	0.01	0.05
High	214	0.08	0.10	282	-0.11	-0.19
Multiple R Squared		0.028	0.094		0.039	0.091
Multiple R		0.168	0.306		0.199	0.302

TABLE 5.16 (cont'd)

able & Category	Thai Muslim (Grand Mean = 3.37)			Southern Thai Muslim (Grand Mean = 3.28)		
	N	Unadjusted Deviation	Adjusted Deviation	N	Unadjusted Deviation	Adjusted Deviation
ehold Types		(0.14)	(0.14)		(0.08)	(0.10)
clear	362	0.29	0.30	406	0.11	0.15
int (one couple)	156	-0.24	-0.32	83	-0.45	-0.40
int (2 or more couples)	93	-0.72	-0.64	69	-0.12	-0.43
Influence		(0.02)	(0.03)		(0.04)	(0.05)
sband	265	0.01	-0.09	369	0.05	0.06
ual	103	-0.11	-0.01	76	-0.23	-0.32
fe	243	0.04	0.10	113	-0.01	0.01
hic Cost of raception		(0.10)	(0.10)		(0.03)	(0.04)
w	83	0.57	0.58	43	0.21	0.27
dium	218	-0.27	-0.23	95	0.08	0.08
gh	310	0.04	0.01	420	-0.04	-0.05
iple R Squared		0.059	0.108		0.034	0.079
iple R		0.242	0.329		0.184	0.281

ACCONT, DFS and FECUN on CEB, RF and UEM. Analysis of variance shows conclusively that current access to contraception is not significantly related to cumulative fertility for all ethnic groups. Desired family size and perceived fecundity are significantly related to fertility for all ethnic groups (Table 5.17).

The results of MCA further show that those who desire a smaller family size average lower fertility than those who desire a large one, implying that motivation to have a smaller family size has a negative impact on actual fertility. The data also show that those who perceive they are not fecund have lower fertility than those who perceive themselves as fecund. The relationship between the two variables may simply reflect the fact that those who have more children naturally perceive that they are generally more fecund than those who have fewer children (Table 5.18).

Model V

Model V focuses on the behaviour of child mortality as it is the only new variable in the model of analysis. Data show that child mortality is a significant factor affecting cumulative fertility of all ethnic groups (Table 5.19). Furthermore, the effects of two-way interaction of child mortality experience, desired family size, and perceived fecundity on children ever born are also significant among the Southern Thai Muslims, implying that child mortality has a stronger effect on cumulative fertility for this ethnic group than for the other ethnic groups.

The MCA results conclusively show that those who have experienced higher child mortality have higher fertility (Table 5.20), implying that fertility reduction can be difficult without reduction in child mortality first as parents would like to be ensured that they have a certain number of surviving children.

Recent Fertility

Model I

Since the Thai Government announced its population policy in early 1971, the Thai people have been exposed to family planning campaigns and have increasingly accepted various fertility

TABLE 5.17

ANOVA of Live Birth: Model IV

Source of Variation	Significance of F				
	Total	Chinese	Thai	Thai Muslim	Southern Thai Muslim
Main Effects	0.000	0.000	0.000	0.000	0.000
Ethnic affiliation (V178)	0.349	0.504	0.012	0.635	0.085
Ethnic fertility approval (V179)	0.000	0.068	0.029	0.074	0.074
Access to contraception (V198)	0.260	0.105	0.595	0.160	0.192
Desired family size (V102)	0.000	0.000	0.000	0.000	0.000
Perceived fecundity (V194)	0.000	0.000	0.000	0.000	0.000
Covariates	0.000	0.000	0.000	0.003	0.010
Couple's income	0.006	0.001	0.516	0.812	0.144
Perceived women's role	0.078	0.043	0.467	0.116	0.244
Religiosity	0.000	0.583	0.032	0.423	0.063
Spouse interaction	0.238	0.387	0.971	0.645	0.294
Months of breastfeeding	0.000	0.000	0.000	0.000	0.007
2-Way Interactions	0.325	0.093	0.854	0.653	0.016
Explained	0.000	0.000	0.000	0.000	0.000
Covariate Raw Regression Coefficient					
Couple's income	0.047	0.067	0.020	0.012	0.099
Perceived women's role	0.088	-0.119	-0.054	0.207	0.165
Religiosity	0.029	-0.008	0.031	0.018	0.079
Spouse interaction	-0.035	-0.039	-0.002	-0.037	-0.088
Months of breastfeeding	0.079	0.190	0.150	0.206	0.113

TABLE 5.18
MCA of Live Birth: Model IV

Variable & Category	Chinese (Grand Mean = 2.87			Thai (Grand Mean = 2.61)		
	N	Unadjusted Deviation	Adjusted Deviation	N	Unadjusted Deviation	Adjusted Deviation
Access to Contraception		(0.08)	(0.04)		(0.01)	(0.03)
Does not know where	121	-0.23	-0.15	127	-0.05	-0.07
More than 30 minutes	69	0.39	0.16	66	-0.03	-0.11
Less than 30 minutes	593	0.00	0.01	638	0.01	0.02
Desired Family Size		(0.66)	(0.63)		(0.70)	(0.67)
0-1 children	201	-1.51	-1.42	315	-1.23	-1.17
3-4 children	437	0.01	-0.01	409	0.22	0.20
Five or more	145	2.07	1.99	107	2.80	2.68
Perceived Fecundity		(0.21)	(0.14)		(0.23)	(0.15)
0 Infecund or difficult	293	-0.47	-0.31	280	-0.59	-0.37
1 Fecund or easy	490	0.28	0.19	551	0.30	0.19
Multiple R Squared		0.462	0.495		0.528	0.549
Multiple R		0.680	0.704		0.727	0.741

TABLE 5.18 (cont'd)

	Thai Muslim (Grand Mean = 2.94)			Southern Thai Muslim (Grand Mean = 2.61)		
Variable & Category	N	Unadjusted Deviation	Adjusted Deviation	N	Unadjusted Deviation	Adjusted Deviation
Access to Contraception		(0.04)	(0.06)		(0.11)	(0.05)
Does not know where	143	-0.14	-0.22	214	0.31	0.12
More than 30 minutes	62	0.25	0.36	45	-0.00	0.11
Less than 30 minutes	397	0.01	0.02	283	-0.23	-0.10
Desired Family Size		(0.52)	(0.47)		(0.59)	(0.55)
0-1 children	162	-0.27	-1.06	165	-0.89	-0.77
3-4 children	269	-0.52	-0.52	219	-0.88	-0.87
Five or more	171	2.02	1.82	158	2.16	2.00
Perceived Fecundity		(0.31)	(0.20)		(0.33)	(0.25)
0 Infecund or difficult	245	-0.95	-0.60	363	-0.54	-0.41
1 Fecund or easy	357	0.65	0.41	179	1.09	0.82
Multiple R Squared		0.333	0.354		0.436	0.451
Multiple R		0.577	0.595		0.660	0.672

TABLE 5.19

ANOVA of Live Birth: Model V

Source of Variation	Significance of F				
	Total	Chinese	Thai	Thai Muslim	Southern Thai Muslim
Main Effects	0.000	0.000	0.000	0.000	0.000
Ethnic affiliation (V178)	0.431	0.885	0.106	0.545	0.404
Ethnic fertility approval (V179)	0.001	0.003	0.558	0.273	0.014
Desired family size (V102)	0.000	0.000	0.000	0.000	0.000
Perceived fecundity (V194)	0.000	0.000	0.000	0.000	0.000
Child mortality experience (V196)	0.000	0.000	0.000	0.000	0.000
Covariates	0.000	0.000	0.000	0.041	0.002
Couple's income	0.000	0.000	0.098	0.274	0.948
Perceived women's role	0.346	0.304	0.933	0.772	0.430
Religiosity	0.585	0.120	0.313	0.854	0.090
Spouse interaction	0.296	0.206	0.999	0.395	0.790
Months of breastfeeding	0.000	0.000	0.000	0.002	0.000

(cont'd on next page)

TABLE 5.19 (cont'd)
ANOVA of Live Birth: Model V

	Significance of F				
Source of Variation	Total	Chinese	Thai	Thai Muslim	Southern Thai Muslim
2-Way Interactions	0.004	0.149	0.500	0.162	0.029
V178 x V179	0.819	0.799	0.475	0.628	0.887
V178 x V102	0.608	0.093	0.461	0.172	0.834
V178 x V194	0.360	0.036	0.459	0.098	0.757
V178 x V196	0.018	0.295	0.140	0.337	0.456
V179 x V102	0.010	0.449	0.991	0.444	0.062
V179 x V194	0.754	0.094	0.091	0.980	0.938
V179 x V196	0.944	0.743	0.678	0.927	0.660
V102 x V194	0.185	0.272	0.202	0.083	0.012
V102 x V196	0.016	0.548	0.125	0.176	0.013
V194 x V196	0.038	0.822	0.259	0.073	0.047
Explained	0.000	0.000	0.000	0.000	0.000
Covariate Raw Regression Coefficient					
Couple's income	0.065	0.075	0.059	0.054	0.005
Perceived women's role	0.049	-0.086	0.007	0.037	0.118
Religiosity	0.005	-0.024	0.016	-0.004	0.079
Spouse interaction	-0.033	-0.058	0.000	-0.067	-0.024
Months of breastfeeding	0.204	0.203	0.181	0.170	0.199

TABLE 5.20
MCA of Live Birth: Model V

Variable & Category	Chinese Grand Mean = 1.89)			Thai (Grand Mean = 1.57)		
	N	Unadjusted Deviation	Adjusted Deviation	N	Unadjusted Deviation	Adjusted Deviation
Desired Family Size		(0.70)	(0.63)		(0.70)	(0.64)
0-1 children	162	-1.50	-1.35	250	-1.20	-1.07
3-4 children	320	0.05	0.03	305	0.20	0.22
Five or more	99	2.28	2.09	77	2.90	2.70
Perceived Fecundity		(0.23)	(0.15)		(0.26)	(0.16)
Infecund or difficult	220	-0.53	-0.34	218	-0.65	-0.41
Fecund or easy	361	0.32	0.21	422	0.34	0.21
Child Mortality Experience		(0.26)	(0.21)		(0.21)	(0.17)
No	526	-0.14	-0.11	574	-0.11	-0.09
One	43	1.22	0.81	50	0.67	0.55
Two or more	12	1.94	1.36	16	2.00	1.62
Multiple R Squared		0.559	0.596		0.557	0.581
Multiple R		0.748	0.772		0.746	0.762

TABLE 5.20 (cont'd)

Variable & Category	Thai Muslim (Grand Mean = 3.29)			Southern Thai Muslim (Grand Mean = 3.16)		
	N	Unadjusted Deviation	Adjusted Deviation	N	Unadjusted Deviation	Adjusted Deviation
Desired Family Size		(0.52)	(0.42)		(0.54)	(0.44)
0-1 children	148	-1.26	-1.26	103	-0.38	-0.33
3-4 children	234	-0.45	-0.38	160	-1.02	-0.82
Five or more	144	2.03	0.65	103	1.96	1.60
Perceived Fecundity		(0.34)	(0.17)		(0.33)	(0.22)
Infecund or difficult	212	-1.02	-0.52	240	-0.56	-0.36
Fecund or easy	314	0.69	0.35	126	1.70	0.69
Child Mortality Experience		(0.44)	(0.33)		(0.48)	(0.35)
No	434	-0.48	-0.36	297	-0.52	-0.37
One	66	1.85	0.31	53	1.80	1.32
Two or more	26	3.37	2.72	16	3.65	2.57
Multiple R Squared		0.441	0.454		0.521	0.545
Multiple R		0.664	0.674		0.722	0.738

regulating or birth control methods. It is, therefore, more appropriate to investigate the pattern of fertility change that has taken place after the promulgation of these population policies. Thus fertility during the last 5 years is an appropriate variable to be investigated.

Analysis of variance shows that among the Chinese, only occupation is significantly related to recent fertility (Table 5.21). For the Thais and the Southern Thai Muslims, husband's education is the only significant variable, and for the Thai Muslims, ethnic fertility approval and husband's education are significant variables, implying the importance of education in determining fertility behaviour for most ethnic groups.

As for the covariates, it has been found that religiosity and length of breastfeeding are significant in all ethnic groups, except among the Southern Thai Muslims where religiosity is not significantly related to recent fertility. For the Thais, the Chinese and the Thai Muslims, religiosity is negatively related to recent fertility, probably due to some recent religious movements which are more tolerant to family planning. No such movement, however, has been found among the Southern Thai Muslims. Breastfeeding practice is also found to be negatively related to recent fertility as it is with cumulative fertility.

The result of multiple classification analysis shows that among the Chinese the level of husband's education in general has a negative effect on recent fertility (Table 5.22). However, when the analysis is controlled for other independent variables and covariates, the relationship between husband's education and recent fertility is curvilinear, and the differences among different educational groups in fertility level become less.

Model II

Similar to the findings on the total number of children ever born, gender balance is significantly related to fertility for all ethnic groups. It is interesting to note the significance of wife's employment to recent fertility among the Thais and the Thai Muslims (Table 5.23). Women who do not work have been found to be more fertile than those who work far away from home and those who work at home, respectively (Table 5.24). The differences in recent fertility among the three groups of women are greater among the Thais than among the Thai Muslims, implying the impact of work is greater among the Thais than among the Thai Muslims and other ethnic groups. This means that a decline in Thai fertility can be effectively induced by encouraging Thai women to participate in the labour force, while a reduction in

TABLE 5.21
ANOVA of Recent Fertility: Model I

	Significance of F				
Source of Variation	Total	Chinese	Thai	Thai Muslim	Southern Thai Muslim
Main Effects	0.035	0.202	0.107	0.016	0.100
Ethnic affiliation (V178)	0.257	0.569	0.738	0.583	0.967
Ethnic fertility approval (V179)	0.131	0.164	0.271	0.047	0.793
Husband's education (V53)	0.227	0.040	0.738	0.590	0.246
Husband's occupation (V75)	0.010	0.462	0.006	0.059	0.006
Wife's education (V55)	0.920	0.964	0.660	0.176	0.238
Covariates	0.000	0.000	0.000	0.000	0.000
Couple's income	0.425	0.131	0.010	0.179	0.091
Perceived women's role	0.322	0.475	0.156	0.197	0.177
Religiosity	0.000	0.002	0.014	0.036	0.286
Spouse interaction	0.758	0.422	0.827	0.677	0.539
Months of breastfeeding	0.000	0.000	0.000	0.000	0.000
2-Way Interactions	0.394	0.698	0.996	0.122	0.743
Explained	0.000	0.000	0.000	0.000	0.000
Covariate Raw Regression Coefficient					
Couple's income	-0.008	0.024	-0.058	-0.032	-0.060
Perceived women's role	0.028	0.044	-0.071	0.078	-0.096
Religiosity	-0.019	-0.035	-0.024	-0.021	-0.023
Spouse interaction	-0.005	-0.027	0.006	0.015	-0.026
Months of breastfeeding	0.159	0.199	0.136	0.170	0.136

TABLE 5.22
MCA of Recent Fertility: Model I

Variable & Category	N	Total (Grand Mean = 0.76) Unadjusted Deviation	Adjusted Deviation
Ethnic Affiliation		(0.02)	(0.04)
Low	802	0.02	0.04
Medium	967	0.01	0.02
High	1,002	-0.02	-0.04
Ethnic Fertility Approval		(0.04)	(0.04)
Scores 1-3	35	-0.16	-0.20
Scores 4-6	1,600	-0.02	-0.02
Scores 7-9	1,136	0.04	0.04
Husband's Education		(0.04)	(0.04)
No schooling or primary	1,680	0.00	-0.03
Some secondary	797	0.03	0.05
Post secondary	294	-0.09	0.00
Husband's Occupation		(0.06)	(0.04)
Professional	1,447	-0.05	-0.04
Services production	881	0.07	0.05
Farm	346	0.04	0.02
Not classified	97	-0.01	-0.00
Wife's Education		(0.02)	(0.02)
No schooling or primary	2,069	0.01	-0.01
Some secondary	556	-0.01	0.03
Post secondary	146	-0.07	0.06
Multiple R Squared		0.007	0.081
Multiple R		0.083	0.285

TABLE 5.22 (cont'd)

Chinese (Grand Mean = 0.79)			Thai (Grand Mean = 0.66)		
N	Unadjusted Deviation	Adjusted Deviation	N	Unadjusted Deviation	Adjusted Deviation
	(0.03)	(0.05)		(0.02)	(0.05)
369	-0.03	-0.05	11	-0.11	-0.15
249	0.05	0.06	349	0.02	0.05
160	-0.01	0.02	496	-0.01	-0.03
	(0.07)	(0.08)		(0.05)	(0.04)
4	0.96	1.04	16	-0.28	-0.21
495	0.00	0.01	549	-0.01	-0.00
279	-0.02	-0.04	264	0.04	0.02
	(0.09)	(0.10)		(0.03)	(0.04)
429	-0.07	-0.09	451	-0.00	-0.03
267	0.12	0.12	282	0.02	0.05
82	-0.01	0.04	96	-0.06	0.01
	(0.06)	(0.05)		(0.12)	(0.10)
586	0.01	0.02	357	-0.10	-0.08
141	-0.04	-0.06	346	0.11	0.09
33	0.21	-0.03	99	-0.04	-0.05
18	-0.24	-0.24	27	0.08	0.13
	(0.02)	(0.01)		(0.02)	(0.09)
560	-0.01	-0.01	612	-0.01	-0.04
187	0.04	0.02	160	0.01	0.07
31	-0.02	-0.01	57	0.06	0.23
	0.017	0.112		0.020	0.096
	0.131	0.334		0.140	0.309

TABLE 5.22 (cont'd)
MCA of Recent Fertility: Model 1

Variable & Category	Thai Muslim (Grand Mean = 0.90)			Southern Thai Muslim (Grand Mean = 0.70)		
	N	Unadjusted Deviation	Adjusted Deviation	N	Unadjusted Deviation	Adjusted Deviation
Ethnic Affiliation		(0.06)	(0.04)		(0.02)	(0.03)
Low	274	-0.04	-0.02	148	-0.02	-0.04
Medium	204	-0.02	-0.01	165	-0.00	-0.00
High	129	0.12	0.07	244	0.01	-0.02
Ethnic Fertility Approval		(0.11)	(0.08)		(0.02)	(0.05)
Scores 1-3	11	-0.36	-0.33	4	-0.20	-0.56
Scores 4-6	317	-0.09	-0.06	239	-0.00	-0.01
Scores 7-9	279	0.12	0.08	314	0.00	0.01
Husband's Education		(0.05)	(0.05)		(0.07)	(0.05)
No schooling or primary	409	0.03	-0.04	391	0.04	0.03
Some secondary	144	-0.03	0.09	104	-0.06	-0.07
Post secondary	54	-0.14	0.04	62	-0.16	-0.06
Husband's Occupation		(0.13)	(0.08)		(0.14)	(0.14)
Professional	299	-0.11	-0.06	205	-0.12	-0.07
Services production	188	0.05	0.01	206	0.17	0.16
Farm	90	0.28	0.18	124	-0.07	-0.15
Not classified	30	-0.00	-0.03	22	0.02	0.02
Wife's Education		(0.09)	(0.04)		(0.06)	(0.08)
No schooling or primary	473	0.05	0.01	424	0.01	-0.04
Some secondary	115	-0.18	-0.07	94	0.05	0.17
Post secondary	19	-0.06	0.11	39	-0.19	0.02
Multiple R Squared		0.035	0.115		0.029	0.108
Multiple R		0.187	0.339		0.171	0.328

TABLE 5.23

ANOVA of Recent Fertility: Model II

Source of Variation	Significance of F				
	Total	Chinese	Thai	Thai Muslim	Southern Thai Muslim
Main Effects	0.000	0.000	0.000	0.000	0.000
Ethnic affiliation (V178)	0.095	0.349	0.306	0.684	0.753
Ethnic fertility approval (V179)	0.456	0.339	0.357	0.238	0.783
Wife's employment (V79)	0.001	0.333	0.003	0.012	0.544
Gender balance (V186)	0.000	0.000	0.000	0.000	0.000
Son preference (V187)	0.088	0.577	0.137	0.079	0.481
Covariates	0.000	0.000	0.000	0.000	0.000
Couple's income	0.864	0.362	0.735	0.485	0.479
Perceived women's role	0.234	0.983	0.428	0.031	0.154
Religiosity	0.000	0.025	0.012	0.010	0.137
Spouse interaction	0.691	0.768	0.587	0.444	0.057
Months of breastfeeding	0.000	0.000	0.000	0.000	0.000
2-Way Interactions	0.312	0.406	0.197	0.041	0.710
Explained	0.000	0.000	0.000	0.000	0.000
Covariate Raw Regression Coefficient					
Couple's income	-0.002	0.018	-0.010	-0.021	-0.035
Perceived women's role	0.039	0.002	-0.044	0.151	-0.118
Religiosity	-0.021	-0.031	-0.027	-0.031	-0.036
Spouse interaction	-0.008	0.012	-0.018	0.033	-0.095
Months of breastfeeding	0.121	0.175	0.095	0.118	0.099

TABLE 5.24
MCA of Recent Fertility: Model II

Variable & Category	Chinese (Grand Mean = 0.75)			Thai (Grand Mean = 0.64)		
	N	Unadjusted Deviation	Adjusted Deviation	N	Unadjusted Deviation	Adjusted Deviation
Wife's Employment		(0.70)	(0.06)		(0.13)	(0.12)
Never worked	93	0.10	0.02	163	0.17	0.15
Work at home	405	-0.03	-0.02	321	-0.06	-0.07
Work far away	20	0.02	0.30	81	-0.12	-0.04
Gender Balance		(0.27)	(0.19)		(0.31)	(0.27)
No children	59	-0.73	-0.51	80	-0.64	-0.54
Balance	151	0.16	0.13	137	0.19	0.20
Imbalance	308	0.06	0.03	348	0.07	0.05
Son Preference		(0.01)	(0.04)		(0.04)	(0.05)
More sons	440	0.00	0.02	402	-0.02	-0.03
More daughters	78	-0.01	-0.09	163	0.06	0.07
Multiple R Squared		0.083	0.147		0.125	0.162
Multiple R		0.289	0.384		0.354	0.403

TABLE 5.24 (cont'd)

Variable & Category	Thai Muslim (Grand Mean = 0.86)			Southern Thai Muslim (Grand Mean = 0.67)		
	N	Unadjusted Deviation	Adjusted Deviation	N	Unadjusted Deviation	Adjusted Deviation
Wife's Employment		(0.14)	(0.12)		(0.02)	(0.05)
Never worked	97	0.25	0.16	175	0.02	0.01
Work at home	254	-0.09	-0.10	151	-0.01	-0.04
Work far away	64	-0.01	0.14	38	-0.01	0.12
Gender Balance		(0.36)	(0.30)		(0.30)	(0.26)
No children	72	-0.80	-0.67	55	-0.63	-0.55
Balance	114	0.20	0.14	117	0.14	0.12
Imbalance	229	0.15	0.14	192	0.10	0.08
Son Preference		(0.06)	(0.07)		(0.02)	(0.03)
More sons	293	-0.04	-0.05	250	-0.01	-0.02
More daughters	112	0.09	0.11	114	0.03	0.03
Multiple R Squared		0.158	0.212		0.096	0.152
Multiple R		0.398	0.460		0.310	0.390

fertility of other ethnic groups may have to be done by some other means.

Model III

Household type is a significant variable affecting recent fertility among the Thais, the Chinese and the Southern Thai Muslims but not among the Thai Muslims in other parts of the country. The data also show that the psychic cost of contraception is significantly related to recent fertility only among the Thai Muslims, probably because they are in the minority in their area (Table 5.25). In such a situation, conformity to the group values and norms, religious or otherwise, is needed for a harmonious life.

It should also be noted that among the Chinese, the overall two-way interaction effects are statistically significant. Specifically, the two-way interactions between household type and ethnic affiliation, ethnic fertility approval and husband's dominance, and household type and psychic cost of contraception, are significantly related to recent fertility, suggesting that the role of psychic cost of contraception and husband's dominance in recent fertility have to be examined in conjunction with other variables. Similarly, among the Thai Muslims, even though only psychic cost of contraception is found to be significantly related to recent fertility, a close examination of the interaction effect shows that the interaction effect of husband's dominance and household type on recent fertility is also significant. Among the Southern Thai Muslims, the interaction effect of household type and husband dominance is significantly related to recent fertility. It should be noted that none of the two-way interactions are significant among the Thais.

The results of Multiple Classification Analysis are interesting (Table 5.26). Those who live in a nuclear household have lower recent fertility than those who live in joint families.

Data also show that among the Thai Muslims, those who feel that they have to pay a higher psychic cost of contraception, due to the pressures of social or religious norms, average higher recent fertility than those who feel the contrary. Even though husband's dominance is not significant in all ethnic groups, the MCA results show that a family in which the wife is more dominant or equal to the husband, has lower recent fertility.

Model IV

Access to contraception is a significant variable for recent fertility among the Chinese but not for the other ethnic groups. Those who do not know where they can get contraception have lower fertility than those who have better contraceptive access (Table 5.27), implying that the former may not feel the need for family planning as they currently have lower fertility than their desired family size.

Analysis of variance also shows that desired family size is related to fertility of the Thais, the Chinese and the Southern Thai Muslims and perceived fecundity is significantly related to recent fertility of all ethnic groups.

The results of MCA further show that those who have 3-4 children have higher recent fertility than those who already have 5 children or more or those who have only 2 children or less, respectively. Probably, those who have 2 children or less are only recently married or have recently planned to have children, and those who have 5 children or more have generally had the number of children they wanted long ago (Table 5.28). The significance of perceived fecundity to recent fertility is nothing more than the statement of the actual relationship between the two variables and needs no further explanation.

Model V

Child mortality experience has a significant effect on recent fertility only among the Southern Thai Muslims (Table 5.29). The overall effect of the two-way interactions of the independent variables are not significant for any ethnic group.

Table 5.30 shows that among the Southern Thai Muslims, those who have experienced higher child mortality show a lower recent fertility than those who have experienced lower child mortality or who have not experienced child mortality at all. It is probable that those with higher child mortality are already those with high cumulative fertility, thus their recent fertility is lower than the fertility of those who have had lower child mortality.

TABLE 5.25

ANOVA of Recent Fertility: Model III

Source of Variation	Significance of F				
	Total	Chinese	Thai	Thai Muslim	Southern Thai Muslim
Main Effects	0.000	0.000	0.108	0.001	0.001
Ethnic affiliation (V178)	0.843	0.625	0.842	0.268	0.922
Ethnic fertility approval (V179)	0.086	0.142	0.172	0.056	0.950
Household type (V49)	0.000	0.000	0.009	0.079	0.000
Wife influence (V193)	0.673	0.089	0.256	0.082	0.295
Psychic cost of contraception (V197)	0.251	0.846	0.972	0.019	0.609
Covariates	0.000	0.000	0.000	0.000	0.000
Couple's income	0.342	0.034	0.018	0.141	0.029
Perceived women's role	0.287	0.163	0.272	0.275	0.150
Religiosity	0.000	0.001	0.004	0.050	0.259
Spouse interaction	0.967	0.474	0.855	0.218	0.578
Months of breastfeeding	0.000	0.000	0.000	0.000	0.000

(cont'd on next page)

TABLE 5.25 (cont'd)

ANOVA of Recent Fertility: Model III

Source of Variation	Significance of F				
	Total	Chinese	Thai	Thai Muslim	Southern Thai Muslim
2-Way Interactions	0.500	0.001	0.395	0.110	0.093
V178 x V179	0.895	0.006	0.159	0.478	0.400
V178 x V49	0.807	0.004	0.378	0.477	0.486
V178 x V193	0.226	0.908	0.427	0.256	0.088
V178 x V197	0.943	0.472	0.535	0.386	0.446
V179 x V49	0.822	0.995	0.444	0.047	0.865
V179 x V193	0.850	0.012	0.219	0.039	0.089
V179 x V197	0.797	0.911	0.650	0.079	0.598
V49 x V193	0.040	0.070	0.627	0.027	0.048
V49 x V197	0.041	0.035	0.087	0.917	0.628
V193 x V197	0.681	0.167	0.380	0.159	0.057
Explained	0.000	0.000	0.000	0.000	0.000
Covariate Raw Regression Coefficient					
Couple's income	-0.009	0.031	-0.050	-0.034	-0.073
Perceived women's role	0.030	0.081	-0.055	0.067	-0.099
Religiosity	-0.021	-0.035	-0.028	-0.020	-0.024
Spouse interaction	-0.001	-0.023	9.005	0.046	-0.023
Months of breastfeeding	0.146	0.162	0.127	0.165	0.122

TABLE 5.26
MCA of Recent Fertility: Model III

Variable & Category	Chinese (Grand Mean = 0.80)			Thai (Grand Mean = 0.67)		
	N	Unadjusted Deviation	Adjusted Deviation	N	Unadjusted Deviation	Adjusted Deviation
Household Types		(0.26)	(0.22)		(0.10)	(0.08)
Nuclear	501	-0.19	-0.15	561	-0.06	-0.05
Joint (one couple)	227	0.28	0.20	197	0.14	0.09
Joint (2 or more couples)	65	0.50	0.47	76	0.09	0.11
Wife Influence		(0.08)	(0.06)		(0.06)	(0.05)
Husband	351	-0.06	-0.05	338	-0.05	-0.04
Equal	126	-0.07	-0.03	152	0.09	0.09
Wife	316	0.10	0.07	344	0.01	-0.00
Psychic Cost of Contraception		(0.01)	(0.04)		(0.01)	(0.01)
Low	227	0.00	0.00	210	0.00	0.02
Medium	352	-0.01	-0.03	312	-0.01	-0.00
High	214	0.01	0.05	282	0.01	-0.01
Multiple R Squared		0.078	0.146		0.018	0.089
Multiple R		0.279	0.382		0.132	0.299

TABLE 5.26 (cont'd)

	Thai Muslim (Grand Mean = 0.91)			Southern Thai Muslim (Grand Mean = 0.70)		
Variable & Category	N	Unadjusted Deviation	Adjusted Deviation	N	Unadjusted Deviation	Adjusted Deviation
Household Types		(0.08)	(0.06)		(0.20)	(0.17)
Nuclear	362	-0.07	-0.05	406	-0.11	-0.09
Joint (one couple)	156	0.13	0.09	83	0.20	0.19
Joint (2 or more couples)	92	0.05	0.04	69	0.40	0.33
Wife Influence		(0.10)	(0.07)		(0.06)	(0.04)
Husband	265	0.08	0.05	369	0.03	0.02
Equal	103	-0.20	-0.14	76	-0.02	0.02
Wife	243	-0.00	0.00	113	-0.09	-0.08
Psychic Cost of Contraception		(0.13)	(0.11)		(0.03)	(0.04)
Low	83	-0.28	-0.26	43	-0.05	-0.00
Medium	218	-0.05	-0.01	95	0.06	0.09
High	310	0.11	0.08	420	-0.01	-0.02
Multiple R Squared		0.044	0.124		0.046	0.117
Multiple R		0.211	0.352		0.216	0.343

TABLE 5.27

ANOVA of Recent Fertility: Model IV

Source of Variation	Significance of F				
	Total	Chinese	Thai	Southern Thai Muslim	Thai Muslim
Main Effects	0.000	0.000	0.000	0.000	0.000
Ethnic affiliation (V178)	0.608	0.559	0.943	0.341	0.954
Ethnic fertility approval (V179)	0.070	0.058	0.319	0.031	0.761
Access to contraception (V198)	0.002	0.004	0.089	0.106	0.264
Desired family size (V102)	0.000	0.000	0.009	0.191	0.003
Perceived fecundity (V194)	0.000	0.011	0.000	0.000	0.000
Covariates	0.000	0.000	0.000	0.000	0.000
Couple's income	0.141	0.043	0.046	0.040	0.026
Perceived women's role	0.321	0.447	0.403	0.236	0.247
Religiosity	0.002	0.001	0.003	0.053	0.535
Spouse interaction	0.574	0.283	0.716	0.596	0.299
Months of breastfeeding	0.000	0.000	0.000	0.000	0.000
2-Way Interactions	0.590	0.415	0.623	0.076	0.398
Explained	0.000	0.000	0.000	0.000	0.000
Covariate Raw Regression Coefficient					
Couple's income	-0.014	-0.031	-0.042	-0.048	-0.076
Perceived women's role	0.028	0.046	-0.041	0.073	-0.103
Religiosity	-0.014	-0.036	-0.029	-0.020	-0.013
Spouse interaction	-0.010	-0.035	0.010	0.020	-0.043
Months of breastfeeding	0.145	0.182	0.129	0.155	0.112

TABLE 5.28

MCA of Recent Fertility: Model IV

Variable & Category	Chinese (Grand Mean = 0.80)			Thai (Grand Mean = 0.67)		
	N	Unadjusted Deviation	Adjusted Deviation	N	Unadjusted Deviation	Adjusted Deviation
Access to Contraception		(0.12)	(0.10)		(0.10)	(0.08)
Does not know where	121	-0.27	-0.23	127	-0.20	-0.16
More than 30 minutes	69	0.11	0.07	66	0.05	0.05
Less than 30 minutes	593	0.04	0.04	638	0.04	0.03
Desired Family Size		(0.14)	(0.14)		(0.10)	(0.10)
0-1 children	201	-0.13	-0.08	315	-0.05	-0.02
3-4 children	437	0.12	0.11	490	0.08	0.07
Five or more	145	-0.20	-0.24	107	-0.14	-0.21
Perceived Fecundity		(0.09)	(0.09)		(0.18)	(0.15)
Infecund or difficult	293	-0.11	-0.11	280	-0.21	-0.18
Fecund or easy	490	0.07	0.07	551	0.11	0.09
Multiple R Squared		0.049	0.135		0.051	0.121
Multiple R		0.220	0.367		0.227	0.348

TABLE 5.28 (cont'd)

MCA of Recent Fertility: Model IV

Variable & Category	Thai Muslim (Grand Mean = 0.91)			Southern Thai Muslim (Grand Mean = 0.70)		
	N	Unadjusted Deviation	Adjusted Deviation	N	Unadjusted Deviation	Adjusted Deviation
Access to Contraception		(0.08)	(0.07)		(0.04)	(0.09)
Does not know where	143	-0.08	-0.07	214	-0.05	-0.10
More than 30 minutes	62	-0.17	-0.15	45	0.03	0.02
Less than 30 minutes	397	0.06	0.05	283	0.03	0.07
Desired Family Size		(0.10)	(0.07)		(0.15)	(0.11)
0-1 children	162	-0.16	-0.11	165	-0.21	-0.15
3-4 children	269	0.05	0.07	219	0.10	0.08
Five or more	171	0.07	-0.01	158	0.09	0.05
Perceived Fecundity		(0.16)	(0.10)		(0.17)	(0.15)
Infecund or difficult	245	-0.19	-0.12	363	-0.11	-0.10
Fecund or easy	357	0.13	0.08	179	0.22	0.20
Multiple R Squared		0.051	0.124		0.054	0.118
Multiple R		0.226	0.352		0.232	0.343

TABLE 5.29

ANOVA of Recent Fertility: Model V

Source of Variation	Significance of F				
	Total	Chinese	Thai	Thai Muslim	Southern Thai Muslim
Main Effects	0.000	0.000	0.000	0.000	0.000
Ethnic affiliation (V178)	0.827	0.367	0.220	0.157	0.997
Ethnic fertility approval (V179)	0.042	0.046	0.545	0.020	0.584
Desired family size (V102)	0.000	0.000	0.000	0.000	0.000
Perceived fecundity (V194)	0.000	0.003	0.000	0.000	0.000
Child mortality experience (V196)	0.130	0.673	0.685	0.515	0.005
Covariates	0.018	0.002	0.061	0.001	0.463
Couple's income	0.051	0.076	0.051	0.003	0.058
Perceived women's role	0.177	0.144	0.901	0.480	0.561
Religiosity	0.016	0.000	0.019	0.194	0.438
Spouse interaction	0.790	0.844	0.826	0.956	0.642
Months of breastfeeding	0.072	0.495	0.636	0.006	0.661
2-Way Interactions	0.193	0.714	0.482	0.461	0.420
Explained	0.000	0.000	0.000	0.000	0.003
Covariate Raw Regression Coefficient					
Couple's income	-0.022	-0.033	-0.049	-0.077	-0.082
Perceived women's role	0.044	0.106	-0.007	0.048	-0.049
Religiosity	-0.013	-0.048	-0.027	-0.015	-0.021
Spouse interaction	-0.005	-0.008	-0.007	0.002	0.024
Months of breastfeeding	0.025	0.020	0.011	0.079	-0.013

TABLE 5.30

MCA of Recent Fertility: Model V

	Chinese (Grand Mean = 1.08)			Thai (Grand Mean = 0.86)		
Variable & Category	N	Unadjusted Deviation	Adjusted Deviation	N	Unadjusted Deviation	Adjusted Deviation
Desired Family Size		(0.20)	(0.21)		(0.14)	(0.14)
0-1 children	162	-0.24	0.22	250	0.12	-0.09
3-4 children	320	0.18	0.19	305	0.13	0.13
Five or more	99	0.19	0.24	77	0.13	-0.21
Perceived Fecundity		(0.12)	(0.12)		(0.22)	(0.21)
Infecund or difficult	220	-0.15	0.16	218	-0.28	-0.26
Fecund or easy	36	0.09	0.10	422	0.14	0.14
Child Mortality Experience		(0.03)	(0.02)		(0.04)	(0.03)
No	526	0.01	0.01	574	0.00	0.00
One	43	-0.05	0.04	50	-0.08	-0.06
Two or more	12	-0.16	0.14	16	0.14	0.10
Multiple R Squared		0.067	0.097		0.078	0.094
Multiple R		0.258	0.311		0.280	0.306

TABLE 5.30 (cont'd)

Variable & Category	Thai Muslim (Grand Mean = 1.50)			Southern Thai Muslim (Grand Mean = 0.70)		
	N	Unadjusted Deviation	Adjusted Deviation	N	Unadjusted Deviation	Adjusted Deviation
Desired Family Size		(0.14)	(0.11)		(0.18)	(0.18)
0-1 children	148	-0.22	-0.17	103	-0.25	-0.24
3-4 children	234	0.06	0.08	160	0.05	0.03
Five or more	144	0.13	0.05	103	0.17	0.20
Perceived Fecundity		(0.17)	(0.13)		(0.21)	(0.22)
Infecund or difficult	212	-0.21	-0.16	240	-0.14	-0.15
Fecund or easy	314	0.14	0.11	126	0.27	0.28
Child Mortality Experience		(0.01)	(0.07)		(0.14)	(0.16)
No	434	0.00	0.03	297	0.03	0.04
One	66	-0.00	-0.11	53	0.04	-0.01
Two or more	26	-0.05	-0.24	16	-0.60	-0.68
Multiple R Squared		0.064	0.100		0.104	0.116
Multiple R		0.254	0.316		0.323	0.340

Use of Effective Method

Model I

Data show that among the Chinese, husband's education is the only significant variable that is related to the use of effective contraception (Tables 5.31 and 5.32). The relationship is, however, curvilinear, probably due to the fact that those who are better educated are also economically better off and so can afford not to practise birth control as compared to those who are somewhat worse off. By contrast, there is a positive relationship between the two variables among the Thais. Those who are better educated practise effective contraception. No variable is found to be significantly related to use of effective method among the Thai Muslims. It is interesting to note that among the Southern Thai Muslims, ethnic affiliation and husband's occupation are the two significant variables.

No influence of the covariates is found to be significant among the Chinese; only months of breastfeeding and couple's income are positively related to use of effective method. Among the Thai Muslims, spouse interaction is negatively related to the dependent variables, and among the Southern Thai Muslims, only religiosity is negatively related to effective contraception. The finding supports an earlier explanation for the negative relationship between fertility and religiosity among the Southern Thai Muslims.

Model II

With respect to the use of effective method(s) of contraception, it has been found that gender balance is significant among the Thais, the Chinese and the Thai Muslims but not for the Southern Thai Muslims (Tables 5.33 and 5.34). It implies that whether or not the three ethnic groups will adopt effective contraception will depend on the sex composition of their children. The data surprisingly show that those whose families do not have a balanced sex composition practice effective contraception more than those who have more balance. Nonetheless, those who have no children practice effective birth control least.

It is interesting to note that wife's employment is significantly related to use of effective contraception only among the Southern Thai Muslims. Those who work at home practise effective contraception less than those who do not work or work far away from home. Women who work far away from home practise

TABLE 5.31

ANOVA of Use of Effective Contraception: Model I

Source of Variation	Significance of F				
	Total	Chinese	Thai	Thai Muslim	Southern Thai Muslim
Main Effects	0.000	0.075	0.145	0.037	0.000
Ethnic affiliation (V178)	0.005	0.139	0.268	0.674	0.025
Ethnic fertility approval (V179)	0.000	0.092	0.431	0.072	0.333
Husband's education (V53)	0.000	0.037	0.041	0.172	0.408
Husband's occupation (V75)	0.000	0.270	0.147	0.288	0.011
Wife's education (V55)	0.848	0.829	0.859	0.695	0.101
Covariates	0.000	0.412	0.012	0.039	0.134
Couple's income	0.000	0.740	0.008	0.117	0.226
Perceived women's role	0.773	0.251	0.225	0.919	0.409
Religiosity	0.000	0.193	0.078	0.301	0.016
Spouse interaction	0.059	0.292	0.607	0.015	0.482
Months of breastfeeding	0.022	0.343	0.047	0.147	0.850
2-Way Interactions	0.511	0.094	0.295	0.786	0.422
Explained	0.000	0.045	0.053	0.210	0.001
Covariate Raw Regression Coefficient					
Couple's income	0.037	0.005	0.060	0.038	-0.041
Perceived women's role	-0.008	-0.064	0.062	-0.006	-0.056
Religiosity	-0.054	0.013	-0.018	-0.011	-0.054
Spouse interaction	-0.033	-0.032	-0.015	-0.090	-0.029
Months of breastfeeding	0.026	0.020	0.040	0.037	-0.004

TABLE 5.32
MCA of Use of Effective Contraception: Model I

Variable & Category	N	Total (Grand Mean = 1.27) Unadjusted Deviation	Adjusted Deviation
Ethnic Affiliation		(0.08)	(0.06)
Low	791	0.01	-0.03
Medium	932	0.09	0.07
High	968	-0.09	-0.04
Ethnic Fertility Approval		(0.12)	(0.08)
Scores 1-3	34	0.29	0.28
Scores 4-6	1,550	0.09	0.06
Scores 7-9	1,107	-0.14	-0.09
Husband's Education		(0.14)	(0.09)
No schooling or primary	1,643	-0.10	-0.07
Some secondary	760	0.18	0.12
Post secondary	288	0.12	0.09
Husband's Occupation		(0.17)	(0.09)
Professional	1,395	0.11	0.04
Services production	862	-0.01	0.03
Farm	340	-0.40	-0.23
Not classified	94	0.01	0.04
Wife's Education		(0.07)	(0.02)
No schooling or primary	2,004	-0.04	-0.01
Some secondary	543	0.12	0.03
Post secondary	144	0.12	0.02
Multiple R Squared		0.054	0.115
Multiple R		0.233	0.339

TABLE 5.32 (cont'd)

Chinese (Grand Mean = 1.53)			Thai (Grand Mean = 1.52)		
N	Unadjusted Deviation	Adjusted Deviation	N	Unadjusted Deviation	Adjusted Deviation
	(0.06)	(0.07)		(0.06)	(0.06)
361	-0.01	-0.02	10	-0.32	-0.31
240	0.07	0.08	336	0.05	0.05
53	-0.08	-0.07	447	-0.03	-0.03
	(0.08)	(0.08)		(0.06)	(0.04)
4	-0.53	-0.56	15	0.14	0.11
79	0.04	0.04	523	0.03	0.02
71	-0.07	-0.07	255	-0.06	-0.05
	(0.08)	(0.09)		(0.08)	(0.09)
18	-0.04	-0.04	435	-0.06	-0.07
55	0.10	0.10	265	0.06	0.06
81	-0.10	-0.12	93	0.12	0.13
	(0.07)	(0.08)		(0.09)	(0.08)
65	-0.01	-0.01	338	0.03	-0.00
38	0.09	0.10	334	0.03	0.05
33	-0.22	-0.22	96	-0.16	-0.11
18	-0.08	-0.11	25	-0.24	-0.26
	(0.01)	(0.02)		(0.03)	(0.03)
42	-0.01	-0.00	582	-0.01	0.01
81	0.01	-0.00	155	0.03	-0.03
31	0.05	0.08	56	0.07	-0.08
	0.024	0.030		0.020	0.038
	0.154	0.174		0.140	0.194

TABLE 5.32 (cont'd)

MCA of Use of Effective Contraception: Model 1

Variable & Category	Thai Muslim (Grand Mean = 1.27) N	Unadjusted Deviation	Adjusted Deviation	Southern Thai Muslim (Grand Mean = 0.53) N	Unadjusted Deviation	Adjusted Deviation
Ethnic Affiliation		(0.04)	(0.04)		(0.18)	(0.12)
Low	723	-0.01	-0.05	147	0.22	0.16
Medium	197	0.05	0.04	159	0.04	0.00
High	129	-0.05	0.03	239	-0.16	-0.10
Ethnic Fertility Approval		(0.10)	(0.09)		(0.05)	(0.06)
Scores 1-3	11	0.55	0.56	4	0.47	0.42
Scores 4-6	313	0.05	0.03	235	0.02	0.04
Scores 7-9	275	-0.08	-0.06	306	-0.03	-0.04
Husband's Education		(0.12)	(0.10)		(0.18)	(0.07)
No schooling or primary	406	-0.08	-0.06	384	-0.09	-0.02
Some secondary	141	0.16	0.14	99	0.13	-0.01
Post secondary	52	0.19	0.14	62	0.36	0.16
Husband's Occupation		(0.12)	(0.06)		(0.20)	(0.15)
Professional	295	0.05	0.01	197	0.18	0.10
Services production	187	-0.01	0.01	203	-0.03	0.01
Farm	87	-0.24	0.12	124	-0.28	-0.22
Not classified	30	0.26	0.19	21	0.23	0.26
Wife's Education		(0.09)	(0.05)		(0.18)	(0.11)
No schooling or primary	467	-0.04	-0.02	413	-0.09	-0.05
Some secondary	113	0.14	0.06	94	0.27	0.18
Post secondary	19	0.26	0.18	38	0.31	0.12
Multiple R Squared		0.034	0.054		0.082	0.097
Multiple R		0.185	0.232		0.287	0.311

TABLE 5.33

ANOVA of Use of Effective Contraception: Model II

Source of Variation	Significance of F				
	Total	Chinese	Thai	Thai Muslim	Southern Thai Muslim
Main Effects	0.000	0.002	0.000	0.002	0.013
Ethnic affiliation (V178)	0.014	0.557	0.681	0.441	0.005
Ethnic fertility approval (V179)	0.000	0.265	0.599	0.200	0.167
Wife's employment (V79)	0.000	0.848	0.058	0.703	0.044
Gender balance (V186)	0.000	0.000	0.000	0.000	0.262
Son preference (V187)	0.035	0.535	0.336	0.918	0.772
Covariates	0.000	0.070	0.006	0.158	0.215
Couple's income	0.000	0.097	0.023	0.292	0.473
Perceived women's role	0.467	0.063	0.150	0.773	0.331
Religiosity	0.000	0.082	0.004	0.352	0.039
Spouse interaction	0.941	0.291	0.479	0.071	0.480
Months of breastfeeding	0.333	0.894	0.880	0.080	0.366

(cont'd on next page)

TABLE 5.33 (cont'd)

ANOVA of Use of Effective Contraception: Model II

Source of Variation	Significance of F				
	Total	Chinese	Thai	Thai Muslim	Southern Thai Muslim
2-Way Interactions	0.527	0.638	0.015	0.610	0.186
V178 x V179	0.272	0.406	0.370	0.908	0.532
V178 x V79	0.930	0.826	0.300	0.589	0.418
V178 x V186	0.934	0.828	0.593	0.486	0.375
V178 x V187	0.962	0.157	0.895	0.163	0.659
V179 x V189	0.588	0.502	0.199	0.754	0.058
V179 x V186	0.705	0.979	0.504	0.684	0.055
V179 x V187	0.410	0.953	0.450	0.800	0.525
V179 x V186	0.557	0.801	0.083	0.304	0.313
V179 x V187	0.131	0.049	0.722	0.426	0.410
V186 x V187	0.011	0.683	0.006	0.106	0.717
Explained	0.000	0.030	0.000	0.045	0.026
Covariate Raw Regression Coefficient					
Couple's income	0.050	0.031	0.072	0.033	0.035
Perceived women's role	-0.025	-0.128	0.084	-0.021	-0.081
Religiosity	-0.055	0.022	-0.032	-0.012	-0.056
Spouse interaction	-0.002	0.040	-0.024	-0.082	0.035
Months of breastfeeding	-0.014	0.004	0.004	-0.058	-0.023

TABLE 5.34

MCA of Use of Effective Contraception: Model II

Variable & Category	Chinese (Grand Mean = 1.51)			Thai (Grand Mean = 1.54)		
	N	Unadjusted Deviation	Adjusted Deviation	N	Unadjusted Deviation	Adjusted Deviation
Wife's Employment		(0.03)	(0.06)		(0.09)	(0.05)
Never worked	92	0.05	0.10	150	-0.11	-0.05
Work at home	388	-0.01	-0.03	304	0.05	0.01
Work far away	20	-0.01	0.09	77	0.06	0.08
Gender Balance		(0.21)	(0.20)		(0.30)	(0.31)
No children	53	-0.51	-0.50	75	-0.59	-0.61
Balance	142	0.00	0.02	135	-0.06	-0.08
Imbalance	289	0.09	0.00	329	0.16	0.17
Son Preference		(0.02)	(0.03)		(0.08)	(0.02)
More sons	426	0.01	0.01	302	0.04	0.01
More daughters	74	-0.05	-0.05	157	-0.10	-0.03
Multiple R Squared		0.052	0.071		0.106	0.133
Multiple R		0.227	0.267		0.325	0.364

(cont'd on next page)

TABLE 5.34 (cont'd)

MCA of Use of Effective Contraception: Model II

Variable & Category	Thai Muslim (Grand Mean = 1.25)			Southern Thai Muslim (Grand Mean = 0.52)		
	N	Unadjusted Deviation	Adjusted Deviation	N	Unadjusted Deviation	Adjusted Deviation
Wife's Employment		(0.05)	(0.01)		(0.13)	(0.13)
Never worked	94	-0.01	-0.01	172	0.02	0.04
Work at home	250	0.03	0.01	149	-0.10	-0.11
Work far away	63	-0.11	-0.02	38	0.27	0.25
Gender Balance		(0.23)	(0.27)		(0.05)	(0.11)
No children	68	-0.48	-0.57	55	0.10	0.23
Balance	114	0.04	0.05	114	0.02	0.03
Imbalance	225	0.13	0.14	190	0.02	0.05
Son Preference		(0.02)	(0.00)		(0.01)	(0.01)
More sons	205	0.01	0.00	245	0.01	0.01
More daughters	122	-0.03	-0.01	114	-0.02	-0.01
Multiple R Squared		0.065	0.083		0.052	0.071
Multiple R		0.254	0.209		0.229	0.267

it more than any other groups, suggesting that there is some relationship between contraceptive practice and work outside the home. It also implies that the rate of family planning practice among the Southern Thai Muslim women can be raised by encouraging them to engage in wage labour outside the confines of the family. However, such encouragement can be implemented in their social context only after a thorough study of their family system.

Model III

Regarding the use of effective contraception, none of the three dependent variables in this model is significant among the Chinese (Tables 5.35 and 5.36). Among the Thais, decision to use effective contraception depends on the type of household a woman lives in, as household type is significantly related to fertility. Among the Southern Thai Muslims and the Thai Muslims in other parts of the country, psychic cost of contraception is significantly related to the use of contraception, implying the strength of socialization among the two ethnic groups. In addition, it has been found that household type and husband's dominance are significant variables among the Thai Muslims but not for the Southern Thai Muslims.

It is interesting to note that among the Thais and the Thai Muslims, those who live in a joint household report they practise effective contraception less than those in a nuclear household even though the findings on cumulative fertility and recent fertility would suggest otherwise. It is possible that those who live in a nuclear household use a family planning method only for spacing purposes and not for limiting their family size, and that those who live in a joint household who have low fertility, both cumulative and recent, may not have achieved the desired number of children yet. Thus fewer practise effective contraception. Among the Thai Muslims, the degree of husband's dominance is curvilinearly related to use of effective contraception.

As for the psychic cost of contraception, the data clearly show that among the Muslims, both in the South and in other parts of the country, those who feel higher psychic cost of contraception practise effective contraception less than those who feel otherwise, suggesting that Muslims are more affected by the psycho-social prohibitions against the use of fertility regulating methods.

Model IV

Access to contraception is significantly related to the dependent

TABLE 5.35

ANOVA of Use of Effective Contraception: Model III

Source of Variation	Significance of F				
	Total	Chinese	Thai	Southern Thai Muslim	Thai Muslim
Main Effects	0.000	0.026	0.014	0.000	0.000
Ethnic affiliation (V178)	0.003	0.298	0.452	0.435	0.001
Ethnic fertility approval (V179)	0.000	0.111	0.456	0.053	0.342
Household type (V49)	0.000	0.219	0.000	0.007	0.352
Wife influence (V193)	0.000	0.098	0.694	0.008	0.163
Psychic cost of contraception (V197)	0.000	0.106	0.382	0.005	0.004
Covariates	0.000	0.410	0.008	0.051	0.236
Couple's income	0.000	0.826	0.003	0.048	0.303
Perceived women's role	0.627	0.244	0.356	0.813	0.511
Religiosity	0.000	0.121	0.030	0.189	0.042
Spouse interaction	0.140	0.408	0.621	0.033	0.933
Months of breastfeeding	0.221	0.404	0.113	0.457	0.241
2-Way Interactions	0.051	0.251	0.064	0.946	0.673
Explained	0.000	0.073	0.002	0.036	0.010
Covariate Raw Regression Coefficient					
Couple's income	0.037	0.003	0.065	0.046	-0.034
Perceived women's role	-0.014	-0.064	0.047	-0.014	-0.045
Religiosity	-0.048	0.015	-0.021	-0.013	-0.046
Spouse interaction	-0.025	-0.025	-0.014	-0.079	-0.003
Months of breastfeeding	0.013	0.018	0.031	0.018	-0.024

TABLE 5.36

MCA of Use of Effective Contraception: Model III

Variable & Category	Chinese (Grand Mean = 1.53)			Thai (Grand Mean = 1.52)		
	N	Unadjusted Deviation	Adjusted Deviation	N	Unadjusted Deviation	Adjusted Deviation
Household Types		(0.06)	(0.07)		(0.14)	(0.14)
Nuclear	483	0.03	0.04	534	0.04	0.04
Joint (one couple)	222	-0.03	-0.05	190	0.03	0.02
Joint (2 or more couples)	64	-0.13	-0.15	75	-0.36	-0.36
Wife Influence		(0.08)	(0.07)		(0.03)	(0.04)
Husband	341	-0.04	-0.03	325	-0.01	-0.03
Equal	119	-0.11	-0.09	144	-0.05	-0.06
Wife	309	0.08	0.07	330	0.01	-0.00
Psychic Cost of Contraception		(0.09)	(0.08)		(0.04)	(0.04)
Scores 0-10	219	0.04	0.03	196	0.03	0.03
Scores 11-13	340	0.05	0.05	330	0.01	0.02
Scores 14-18	210	-0.12	-0.11	273	-0.04	-0.05
Multiple R Squared		0.026	0.033		0.027	0.043
Multiple R		0.162	0.181		0.164	0.213

(cont'd on next page)

TABLE 5.36 (cont'd)

MCA of Use of Effective Contraception: Model III

Variable & Category	Thai Muslim (Grand Mean = 1.72)			Southern Thai Muslim (Grand Mean = 1.53)		
	N	Unadjusted Deviation	Adjusted Deviation	N	Unadjusted Deviation	Adjusted Deviation
Household Types		(0.13)	(0.13)		(0.10)	(0.07)
Nuclear	356	0.05	0.05	394	-0.02	-0.03
Joint (one couple)	155	0.06	0.05	83	0.20	0.14
Joint (2 or more couples)	92	-0.29	-0.29	69	-0.11	-0.01
Wife Influence		(0.12)	(0.11)		(0.09)	(0.08)
Husband	259	-0.09	-0.06	361	-0.00	0.02
Equal	103	-0.11	-0.15	72	0.17	0.11
Wife	241	0.15	0.13	113	-0.09	-0.12
Psychic Cost of Contraception		(0.14)	(0.13)		(0.15)	(0.14)
Scores 0-10	82	0.21	0.22	41	0.35	0.34
Scores 11-13	212	0.10	0.08	92	0.15	0.14
Scores 14-18	309	-0.13	-0.11	413	-0.07	-0.07
Multiple R Squared		0.061	0.079		0.066	0.078
Multiple R		0.248	0.202		0.257	0.279

variable (for all ethnic groups) (Table 5.37), whereas desired family size is significant only among the Chinese, and perceived fecundity is significant among the Chinese and the Thais. The two-way interaction effects are not significant for all ethnic groups.

Model V

With respect to the use of effective contraception, analysis of variance shows that child mortality by itself is not significantly related to the dependent variable for all ethnic groups. However, the effect of its interaction effect with ethnic affiliation is significant among the Thais. The interaction effect of child mortality and desired family size is significant among the Chinese (Table 5.39).

The MCA result shows that those who have experienced higher child mortality practise effective contraception less than those who have experienced lower child mortality (Table 5.40). However, the differences among them are too small to be significant for all ethnic groups.

Path Analysis

The results of analysis of variance and multiple classification analysis presented above have been restricted in presenting an overview of the relationships of all the variables of interest. The technique of path analysis enables us to do so by ordering all the variables involved according to the theoretical framework outlined in Chapter I.

There are three models of path analysis: one for cumulative fertility, one for recent fertility and one for use of effective contraception. Diagram 5.1 shows that the result of path analysis of cumulative fertility generally confirms the hypotheses presented in Chapter I; that is, women who are strongly affiliated with their own ethnic group are less educated than those who are not. Those who belong to an older cohort are less educated than those who belong to a younger cohort. A woman's education, in turn, is positively related to her employment outside home. Her employment is negatively related to husband's dominance and positively related to couple's income, which is, in turn, negatively related to religiosity and child mortality experience. Husband's dominance is positively related to son preference which is, in turn, positively related to desired family size and cumulative fertility. Desired family size is also found to be negatively related to age at first marriage and ethnic fertility approval, and positively to months of breastfeeding, child mortality experience, and psychic cost of contraception. Ethnic fertility approval, negatively related to desired family size, is found to be negatively related to religiosity and positively related to woman's education. With respect to husband's occupation, which is a set of three dummy variables, those who are involved in a professional occupation earn a higher income than those who are engaged in farming. The professional workers are also less dominant in interactions with their wives than the farmers.

Diagram 5.2 which treats recent fertility as the final dependent variable has added contraceptive practice as a dependent variable of psychic cost of contraception. Desired family size remains as one of the determinants of recent fertility. The data show that practice of contraception is negatively affected by psychic cost of contraception but positively related to recent fertility. The positive relationship between recent fertility and use of contraception suggests that recent fertility is the independent variable of contraceptive practice.

Diagram 5.3 treats contraceptive practice as the final dependent variable. Analysis of data shows that contraceptive practice is negatively related to months of breastfeeding and positively related to age at first marriage. That is to say, those who married at an older age practice contraception more than those who married at a younger age. Those women who are poorer and who breastfeed their children longer practise family planning less than those whose who breastfeed their children for a shorter duration.

Stepwise Regression Analysis by Ethnic Group

Because unequal sampling fractions were used in drawing the four ethnic groups from their populations, biased results would probably occur in the analysis of data that treats the four groups as if they were randomly drawn from the populations with equal probability of selection. One way to avoid the problem is to apply appropriate use of multiple regression analysis. Another way is to use analysis of variance because its statistical design is appropriate for the stratified sample design.

The analysis of variance used jointly with multiple classification analysis helps identify the form of relationships

TABLE 5.37

ANOVA of Use of Effective Contraception: Model IV

Source of Variation	Significance of F				
	Total	Chinese	Thai	Southern Thai Muslim	Thai Muslim
Main Effects	0.000	0.000	0.000	0.000	0.000
Ethnic affiliation (V178)	0.016	0.416	0.516	0.836	0.000
Ethnic fertility approval (V179)	0.000	0.210	0.138	0.018	0.497
Access to contraception (V198)	0.000	0.000	0.000	0.000	0.000
Desired family size (V102)	0.000	0.027	0.144	0.843	0.838
Perceived fecundity (V194)	0.000	0.001	0.000	0.326	0.282
Covariates	0.000	0.575	0.002	0.443	0.101
Couple's income	0.000	0.626	0.000	0.174	0.104
Perceived women's role	0.925	0.277	0.103	0.937	0.412
Religiosity	0.000	0.0325	0.081	0.461	0.035
Spouse interaction	0.030	0.179	0.609	0.135	0.411
Months of breastfeeding	0.941	0.991	0.241	0.865	0.548
2-Way Interactions	0.236	0.068	0.378	0.487	0.251
Explained	0.000	0.000	0.000	0.000	0.000
Covariate Raw Regression Coefficient					
Couple's income	0.034	0.007	0.075	0.028	-0.052
Perceived women's role	-0.003	-0.058	0.080	-0.004	-0.055
Religiosity	-0.042	-0.009	-0.017	-0.007	-0.046
Spouse interaction	-0.035	0.040	-0.014	-0.050	-0.033
Months of breastfeeding	-0.001	-0.000	-0.022	-0.004	-0.012

TABLE 5.38

MCA of Use of Effective Contraception: Model IV

Variable & Category	Chinese (Grand Mean = 1.52)			Thai (Grand Mean = 0.53)		
	N	Unadjusted Deviation	Adjusted Deviation	N	Unadjusted Deviation	Adjusted Deviation
Access to Contraception		(0.18)	(0.16)		(0.22)	(0.19)
Does not know where	111	-0.37	-0.33	120	-0.43	-0.38
More than 30 minutes	64	0.17	0.10	63	0.03	0.04
Less than 30 minutes	585	0.05	0.05	612	0.08	0.07
Desired Family Size		(0.10)	(0.09)		(0.07)	(0.06)
0-1 children	196	-0.11	-0.09	305	-0.08	-0.06
3-4 children	423	0.08	0.07	392	0.05	0.04
Five or more	141	-0.08	-0.09	98	0.05	0.03
Perceived Fecundity		(0.14)	(0.12)		(0.24)	(0.24)
Infecund or difficult	284	-0.15	-0.13	271	-0.28	-0.28
Fecund or easy	428	0.09	0.08	524	0.15	0.14
Multiple R Squared		0.063	0.068		0.108	0.129
Multiple R		0.252	0.261		0.329	0.360

TABLE 5.38 (cont'd)

	Thai Muslim (Grand Mean = 1.28)			Southern Thai Muslim (Grand Mean = 0.53)		
Variable & Category	N	Unadjusted Deviation	Adjusted Deviation	N	Unadjusted Deviation	Adjusted Deviation
Access to Contraception		(0.46)	(0.45)		(0.34)	(0.35)
Does not know where	140	-0.78	-0.76	209	-0.36	-0.38
More than 30 minutes	60	0.45	0.46	45	0.25	0.25
Less than 30 minutes	394	0.21	0.20	276	0.23	0.24
Desired Family Size		(0.06)	(0.03)		(0.04)	(0.02)
0-1 children	159	-0.05	-0.04	162	0.04	0.03
3-4 children	267	0.07	0.02	215	0.01	0.01
Five or more	168	-0.06	0.00	153	-0.05	-0.02
Perceived Fecundity		(0.02)	(0.04)		(0.02)	(0.04)
Infecund or difficult	242	-0.02	-0.05	354	0.01	-0.03
Fecund or easy	352	0.02	0.03	176	-0.03	0.05
Multiple R Squared		0.227	0.233		0.149	0.164
Multiple R		0.476	0.483		0.386	0.404

TABLE 5.39

ANOVA of Use of Effective Contraception: Model V

Source of Variation	Significance of F				
	Total	Chinese	Thai	Thai Muslim	Southern Thai Muslim
Main Effects	0.000	0.004	0.000	0.086	0.150
Ethnic affiliation (V178)	0.002	0.268	0.361	0.331	0.007
Ethnic fertility approval (V179)	0.000	0.246	0.474	0.081	0.626
Desired family size (V102)	0.000	0.025	0.212	0.240	0.421
Perceived fecundity (V194)	0.000	0.004	0.000	0.675	0.519
Child mortality experience (V196)	0.010	0.743	0.193	0.166	0.946
Covariates	0.000	0.604	0.003	0.028	0.228
Couple's income	0.000	0.969	0.001	0.041	0.664
Perceived women's role	0.444	0.307	0.214	0.971	0.679
Religiosity	0.000	0.493	0.119	0.315	0.063
Spouse interaction	0.214	0.223	0.605	0.035	0.477
Months of breastfeeding	0.187	0.348	0.032	0.095	0.107

(cont'd on next page)

TABLE 5.39 (cont'd)

ANOVA of Use of Effective Contraception: Model V

Source of Variation	Significance of F				
	Total	Chinese	Thai	Thai Muslim	Southern Thai Muslim
2-Way Interactions	0.635	0.022	0.100	0.493	0.578
V178 x V179	0.293	0.266	0.236	0.670	0.481
V178 x V102	0.315	0.051	0.363	0.883	0.875
V178 x V194	0.477	0.059	0.497	0.054	0.191
V178 x V196	0.197	0.221	0.016	0.542	0.165
V179 x V102	0.757	0.066	0.644	0.727	0.936
V179 x V194	0.667	0.032	0.833	0.813	0.693
V169 x V196	0.938	0.330	0.739	0.477	0.215
V102 x V194	0.581	0.215	0.096	0.540	0.794
V102 x V196	0.419	0.252	0.061	0.016	0.693
V194 x V196	0.624	0.905	0.432	0.883	0.814
Explained	0.000	0.003	0.000	0.095	0.315
Covariate Raw Regression Coefficient					
Couple's income	0.048	-0.001	0.082	0.052	0.019
Perceived women's role	-0.024	-0.064	0.073	0.002	-0.035
Religiosity	-0.044	0.008	-0.018	-0.011	-0.049
Spouse interaction	-0.024	-0.042	-0.017	-0.084	0.037
Months of breastfeeding	0.018	0.023	0.049	0.047	-0.048

TABLE 5.40

MCA of Use of Effective Contraception: Model V

	Chinese (Grand Mean = 1.51)			Thai (Grand Mean = 1.49)		
Variable & Category	N	Unadjusted Deviation	Adjusted Deviation	N	Unadjusted Deviation	Adjusted Deviation
Desired Family Size		(0.12)	(0.10)		(0.08)	(0.05)
0-1 children	160	-0.14	-0.12	250	-0.09	-0.05
3-4 children	313	0.09	0.08	296	0.05	0.04
Five or more	97	-0.05	-0.07	73	0.08	0.00
Perceived Fecundity		(0.14)	(0.12)		(0.25)	(0.26)
Infecund or difficult	216	-0.15	-0.14	211	-0.30	-0.31
Fecund or easy	351	0.09	0.08	408	0.16	0.16
Child Mortality Experience		(0.05)	(0.03)		(0.07)	(0.07)
No	516	-0.01	-0.01	556	0.01	0.01
One	42	0.11	0.06	48	-0.20	-0.19
Two or more	12	0.16	0.13	15	0.11	0.13
Multiple R Squared		0.041	0.047		0.078	0.105
Multiple R		0.203	0.218		0.279	0.323

TABLE 5.40 (cont'd)

Variable & Category	Thai Muslim (Grand Mean = 1.26)			Southern Thai Muslim (Grand Mean = 0.75)		
	N	Unadjusted Deviation	Adjusted Deviation	N	Unadjusted Deviation	Adjusted Deviation
Desired Family Size		(0.09)	(0.08)		(0.07)	(0.05)
0-1 children	147	-0.05	-0.07	103	0.06	0.05
3-4 children	232	0.09	0.08	157	0.02	0.01
Five or more	141	-0.09	-0.06	100	-0.10	-0.07
Perceived Fecundity		(0.00)	(0.02)		(0.01)	(0.04)
Infecund or difficult	210	0.00	-0.02	235	0.00	-0.03
Fecund or easy	310	-0.00	0.01	125	-0.01	0.05
Child Mortality Experience		(0.09)	(0.09)		(0.03)	(0.01)
No	428	0.04	0.04	291	0.01	-0.00
One	66	-0.16	-0.13	53	-0.02	0.01
Two or more	26	-0.26	-0.26	16	-0.13	-0.01
Multiple R Squared		0.029	0.053		0.037	0.056
Multiple R		0.170	0.229		0.192	0.257

FIGURE 5.1

Path Model of Ethnicity, Socio-Economic Variables, and Cumulative Fertility

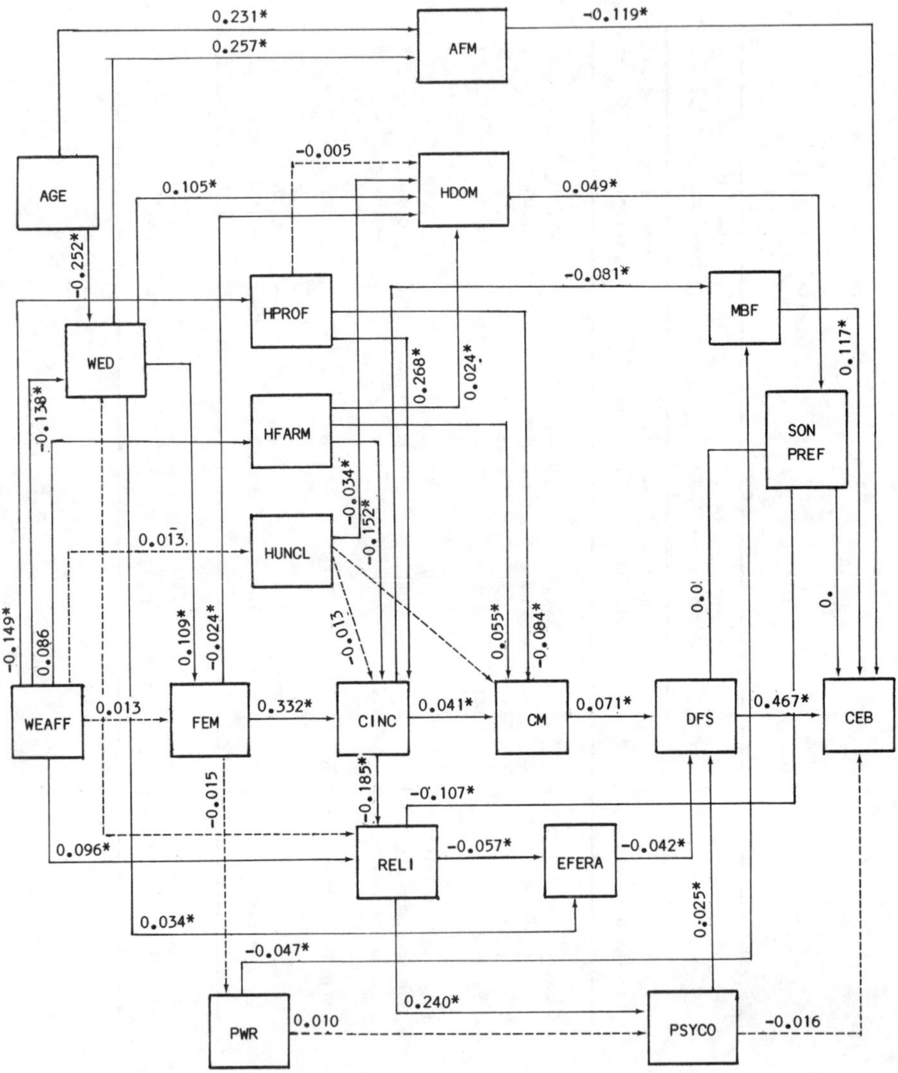

NOTE: * significant at least at .05.
--- hypothesized but not statistically significant.

FIGURE 5.2

Path Model of Ethnicity, Socio-Economic Variables, and Recent Fertility

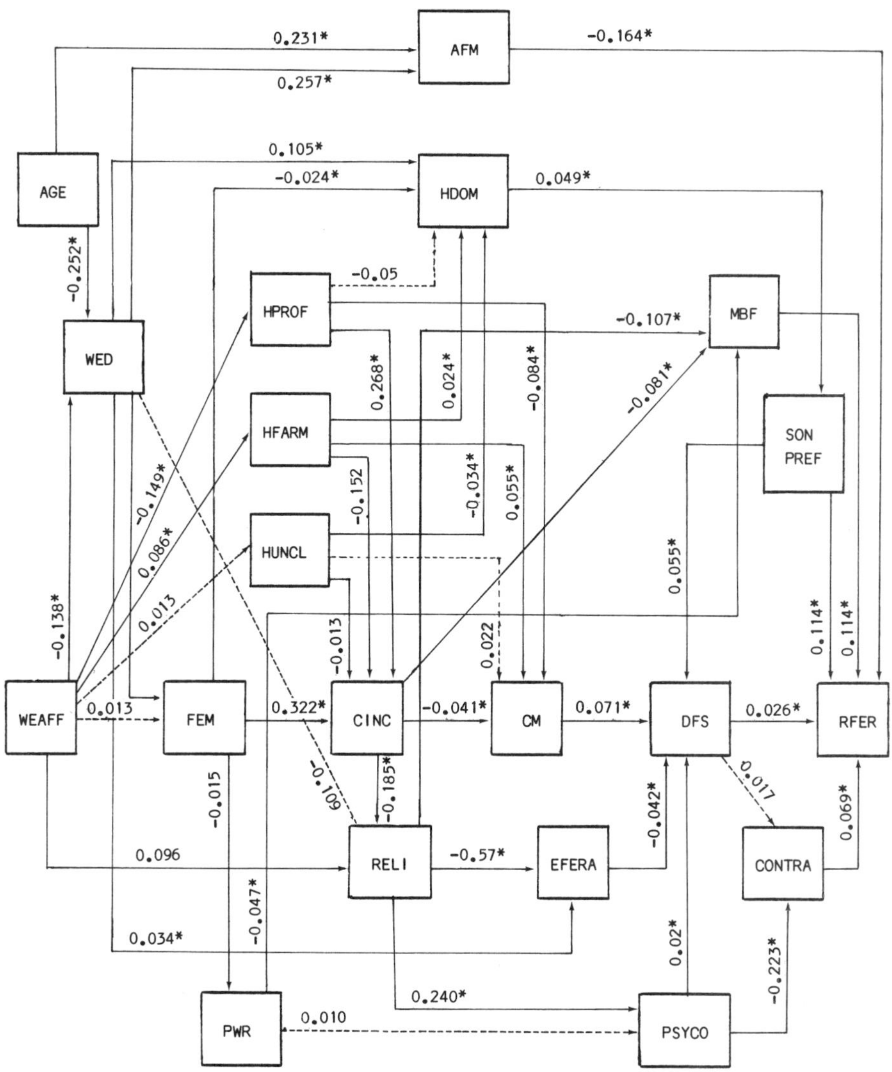

NOTE: * significant at least at .05.

--- hypothesized but not statistically significant.

FIGURE 5.3

Path Model of Ethnicity, Socio-Economic Variables, and Contraception

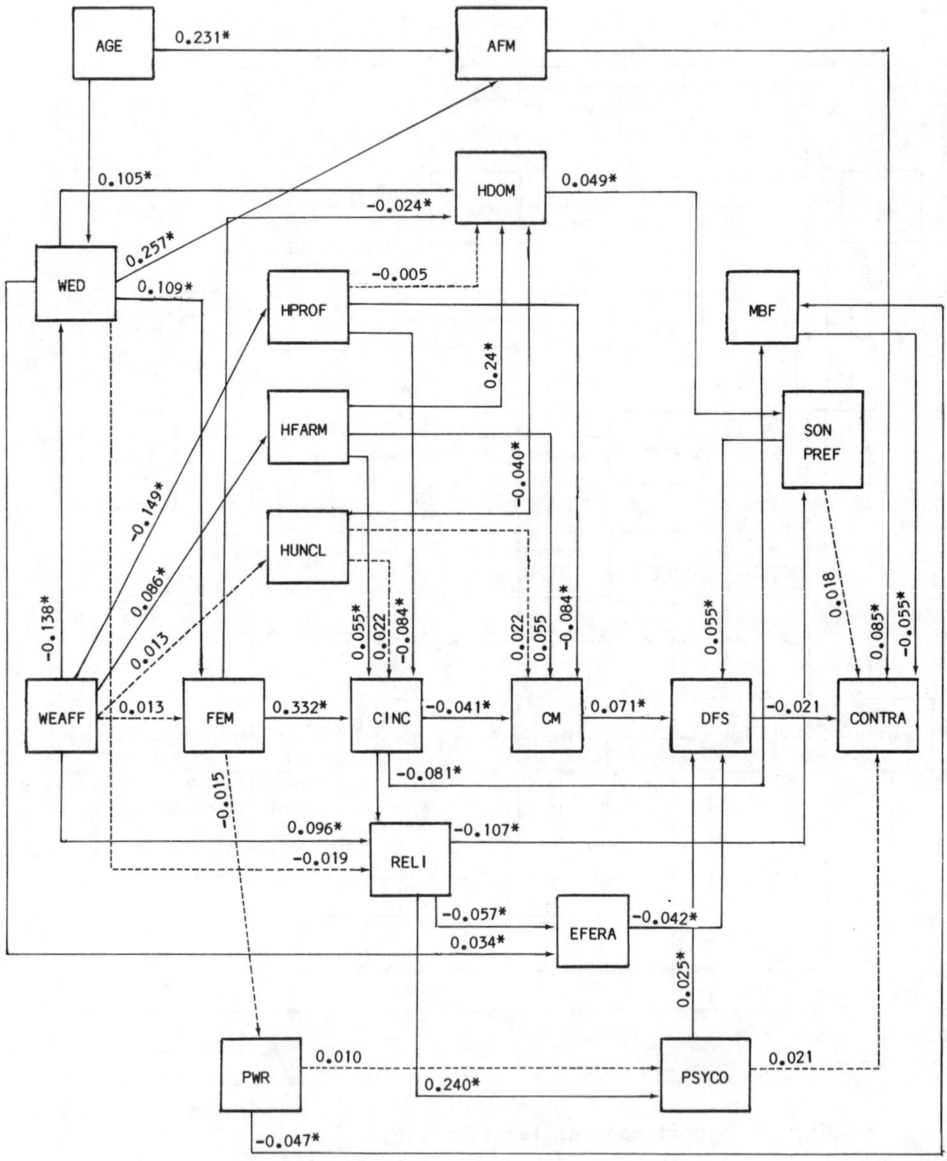

NOTE: * significant at least at .05.

--- hypothesized but not statistically significant.

between the dependent and the independent variables. However, the available analysis of variance (ANOVA) programme has two basic limitations: (1) it can analyse only the main and the interaction effects of the independent and covariate variables and (2) the available ANOVA computer program allows for only five independent variables and five covariates.

Because of the many independent variables to be handled by the available analysis of variance programme, the need to make an estimate of the values of the dependent variable(s), and the nature of the sample design, we need to use multiple regression analysis, which takes the sample design into consideration. This method is one of the most effective ways to analyse the effect of ethnicity on fertility.

To avoid the problem of stratified sampling, multiple regression analysis is done by ethnic group. To derive the most appropriate model for each ethnic group which includes only the significant variables, stepwise analysis is used. The derived models will be used to make estimates of the values of the dependent variables adjusted for the differences in the means of the independent variables among the ethnic groups.

Table 5.41 presents the means and standard deviations of all the variables used in the multiple regression analysis by ethnic group. An examination of the matrices of simple correlation coefficients of all ethnic groups shows that the independent variables remaining in the multiple regression models are not strongly correlated with one another*.

Regression Analysis of Fertility by Ethnic Group

Table 5.42 shows the regression equations for estimating the (adjusted) means of the number of children ever born by ethnic group. Analysis shows that desired family size, marriage duration, gender balance and perceived fecundity are significant variables that commonly affect the cumulative fertility of the four ethnic groups. Even though the significance of the four variables on cumulative fertility is self-explanatory, it is interesting to note that gender balance of living children is a major factor affecting fertility of all ethnic groups, implying

---

* The matrices of simple coorelation coefficients are shown in Appendices A.1 - A.4.

TABLE 5.41

Means and Standard Deviations of All Variables Used in Regression Analysis of CEB, RF, and UEM by Ethnic Group

Variable	Thai	
	$\bar{X}$	S.D
V82 Children ever born	2.62	1.8
V176 Recent fertility	0.66	0.8
V115 Use of effective contraception	1.52	0.8
V178 Ethnic affiliation	4.08	1.0
V179 Ethnic fertility approval	2.29	0.5
V53 Husband's education	1.63	1.0
V75 Husband's occupation	0.12	0.3
V183 Grouped couple's income	1.38	1.3
V55 Wife's education	1.29	0.6
V79 Wife's employment	0.88	0.6
V184 Perceived woman's role	1.76	0.5
V185 Religiosity	11.57	2.9
V186 Gender balance	1.95	1.0
V187 Son preference	0.36	0.4
V49 Types of household	0.68	0.4
V192 Spouse interaction	3.13	1.0
V193 Wife's influence	0.41	0.4
V197 Psychic cost of contraception	3.13	0.9
V198 Access to contraception	0.96	0.6
V102 Desired family size	3.04	1.3
V194 Perceived fecundity	0.67	0.5
V195 Months of breastfeeding	1.43	1.5
V196 Child mortality experience	2.19	3.7
V51 Years of urban residence	12.80	15.3
V152 Age at first marriage	21.91	4.4
V180 Marriage duration	10.81	7.0

TABLE 5.41 (cont'd)

Chinese		Thai Muslim		Southern Thai Muslim	
X̄	S.D	X̄	S.D	X̄	S.D
2.92	1.84	3.24	2.54	3.25	2.47
0.80	0.99	0.77	0.98	0.69	0.90
1.51	0.85	1.27	0.95	0.52	0.86
2.67	1.13	2.59	1.32	3.21	1.27
2.32	0.60	2.41	0.61	2.56	0.69
1.65	1.30	1.45	0.95	1.22	0.93
0.04	0.20	0.13	0.34	0.23	0.42
2.84	2.25	1.77	1.70	0.82	1.12
1.27	0.63	1.19	0.59	1.03	0.85
0.87	0.60	0.87	0.70	0.67	0.67
1.78	0.56	2.25	0.65	1.73	0.54
0.02	3.76	13.40	3.72	17.10	1.75
2.01	0.91	1.69	1.10	1.95	1.02
0.21	0.41	0.33	0.47	0.34	0.47
0.63	0.48	0.60	0.49	0.73	0.45
3.01	1.03	3.09	1.04	3.07	0.91
0.40	0.49	0.38	0.48	1.20	0.40
3.02	0.92	3.56	1.00	3.98	1.02
0.98	0.68	0.89	0.77	0.75	0.82
3.35	1.40	3.54	1.71	3.36	1.99
0.63	0.48	0.58	0.49	0.32	0.47
1.26	1.46	1.39	1.57	1.43	1.84
2.40	3.90	1.48	3.14	3.14	4.15
3.75	16.01	14.64	16.14	11.74	14.90
3.44	4.52	21.36	4.69	19.60	4.87
1.43	7.20	10.86	7.56	12.75	8.53

TABLE 5.42
Regression Equations for Estimating Mean and Adjusted Mean of Children Ever Born

Variable	Thai	Chinese	Thai Muslim	Southern Thai Muslim
V.51 YUR				+0.026 (3)
V.55 WED		-0.144*	-0.303 (5)	
V1.02 DFS	+0.556 (2)	+0.404 (2)	+0.260 (3)	+0.192 (4)
V.152 AFM		-0.025 (5)		
V.179 EFERA			+0.288 (6)	
V.180 MD	+0.124 (1)	+0.130 (1)	+0.198 (1)	+0.172 (1)
V.183 CINC	+0.066*(5)			
V.186 GENB	+0.176 (4)	+0.352 (3)	+0.183 (4)	+0.221 (5)
V.194 PF	+0.411 (3)	+0.520 (4)	+0.922 (2)	+1.296 (2)
V.195 MBF	+0.055*(6)			
Constant	-1.012	-0.172	-1.008	-0.738
Adjusted R^2	0.648	+0.648	+0.579	0.614
Standard error	1.109	+1.094	+1.647	1.538
Original mean	2.62	2.93	3.24	3.26
Adjusted mean				
Thai	2.62	2.76	3.17	3.34
Chinese	2.76	2.93	3.35	3.48
Thai Muslim	2.80	2.86	3.24	3.31
Southern Thai Muslim	2.94	3.06	3.47	3.26

NOTES: In the parentheses is the order of inclusion of the variable(s) in the equation(s). The asterisked variables are significant at .05 and the non-asterisked ones are significant at .01 level of significance.

all ethnic groups attempt to achieve some balance in the sex composition of their children. Such an attempt has a positive impact on their fertility.

Analysis of the data also shows that fertility of each ethnic group is also affected by other variables. Among the Thais, couple's income and months of breastfeeding are positively related to fertility. The positive correlation between month of breastfeeding and fertility is probably due to the fact that breastfeeding is generally practised by lower socio-economic groups and the analysis has not adequately controlled for it, despite a large number of variables included in the analysis.

Among the Chinese, it is significant that wife's education and age at first marriage are negatively related to fertility. This implies that Chinese women who are better educated and who married at an older age tend to have lower fertility than those who are less educated and who married at a younger age. Even though the results are generally expected, they at least significantly modify, if not rule out, the generalization that the Chinese in Thailand tend to have large families. In fact, family size depends on a number of social and economic factors.

The data also show that fertility of the Thai Muslims is also affected by other variables such as wife's education and ethnic fertility approval. While education negatively affects their fertility, ethnic fertility approval is found to affect it positively. The net effect of all the variables that are significantly related to Thai Muslim fertility is a higher level of fertility among the Thai Muslims compared with the Thais and the Chinese, as shown in their respective means.

Insofar as the Southern Thai Muslims are concerned, all the factors that are found to be significantly related to their fertility are positively related to it. In addition to the four variables that significantly affect fertility of all ethnic groups, years of urban residence is found to be another variable that is significantly related to the Southern Thai Muslim. The positive coefficient is not expected but can be readily explained by the fact that the urban Southern Thai Muslims are generally in a better position to have larger families than those who live in the rural areas.

The analysis so far has focused on factors affecting fertility of each ethnic group. In order to derive the net effect of ethnicity on fertility, the assumption has to be made that the fertility of an ethnic group is affected by the same set of variables as that of the other group(s).

Based on this assumption, the net effect of ethnicity on

fertility is assessed by applying the mean values of the variables (found to be significant in an equation) of each ethnic group to the equation. For instance, when the regression equation of the Thai sample is used as the criterion, the mean values of the variables of another ethnic group, say the Chinese, are applied to the equation to estimate the mean of the dependent variable. The difference between the original mean value of the dependent variable and the estimated mean (based on the mean values of the independent variable of other ethnic group[s]) reflects the net effect of ethnicity, e.g., being Chinese, on fertility. Other equations can take turns being the criteria.

Table 5.42 shows that the Thais have a lower fertility (2.62 children) than the Chinese (2.93), the Thai Muslims (3.24), and the Southern Thai Muslims (3.26). If the Thais were to have the same characteristics as other ethnic groups, their fertility would still be lower than the other ethnic groups, shown in the Thai column of the lower portion of Table 5.42.

Read vertically, every column (of the bottom portion) of the Table shows that while the Thais have lowest fertility, the Southern Thai Muslims' fertility is highest, except when other ethnic groups accept the significance of the variables of the Southern Thai Muslims (when using the Southern Thai Muslim equation). The results imply that (i) the Thais and the Chinese generally have lower fertility than the Southern Thai Muslims; (ii) fertility of the Southern Thai Muslims would be lower if their fertility was affected by the same set of independent variables of the Thai and Chinese groups. If the Southern Thai Muslims, with their own variable means, behaved like other ethnic groups (by letting their fertility be affected by the same set of variables that affect the fertility of other ethnic groups), their fertility would be lower.

The data also show that the Thai Muslims generally tend to have higher fertility than the Thais and lower fertility than the Southern Thai Muslims. But the Thai Muslims can have lower or higher fertility than the Chinese, depending on the equations used as the criterion. The Muslim groups would have a higher fertility than the Chinese if their fertility was affected by the Thai set of variables and a lower fertility than the Chinese if their fertility was affected by the set of variables of the other ethnic groups. The results imply that the Thai Muslims in general have higher fertility than the Thais and the Chinese. However their fertility would be lower if their fertility were affected by the sets of variables that affected fertility of the Thais and the Chinese.

In brief, analysis of data shows that there are significant ethnic fertility differentials and that each ethnic group is affected by a common set of factors as well as by other factors that are unique to each ethnic group. This implies that while a common programme can be applied to all ethnic groups, a programme designed to take care of the unique characteristics of each ethnic group is also necessary.

Regression Analysis of Effective Contraception by Ethnic Group

Table 5.43 shows the regression equations for estimating the (adjusted) means of effective contraception by ethnic group. Data show that the Thais use more effective contraception (an average score of 1.55) than the Chinese (1.51), the Thai Muslims (1.27) and the Southern Thai Muslims (.52) and that access to contraception is a positive factor that affects the use of contraception to all ethnic groups.

Among the Thais, all the factors that significantly affect their use of effective contraception are found to be positive. The significant factors are couple's income, perceived woman's role, gender balance, perceived fecundity, household type, and access to contraception. The findings imply that those who are more modern in their attitude towards the woman's role, earn a higher income, live in a nuclear household, have high perceived fecundity, have a gender balance in terms of children's composition and access to contraception, tend to use more effective methods of birth control than those who have the opposite characteristics.

The use of effective contraception by the Chinese is positively influenced by gender balance, perceived fecundity and access to contraception and negatively affected by husband's professional occupation. The latter is probably due to the fact that those who are in professional occupations are better off than those who are not and consequently do not feel compelled to use effective contraception. The same variable similarly affects the contraceptive behaviour of the Thai Muslims and the Southern Thai Muslims.

Among the Thai Muslims, use of effective contraception is positively affected by access to contraception, wife's influence and gender balance, and negatively affected by husband's professional occupation, wife's ethnic fertility approval and psychic cost of using contraception. The negative correlation between ethnic fertility approval and use of effective contraception implies that those who disapprove of high fertility among their own ethnic group members tend to use effective

TABLE 5.43
Regression Equations for Estimating Mean and Adjusted Means of Effective Contraception Score

Variable	Thai	Chinese	Thai Muslim	Southern Thai Muslim
V.49 HTYPE	+0.126*(6)			
V.55 WED				+0.126 (2)
V.75 HOCC		-0.347*(4)	-0.243 (3)	-0.183*(6)
V.178 WEAFF				-0.075 (3)
V.179 EFERA			-0.118*(6)	
V.183 CINC	+0.064 (3)			
V.184 PWR	+0,103*(5)			
V.185 RELI				-0.044*(5)
V.186 GENB	+0.121 (2)	+0.086 (3)	+0.085 (4)	
V.193 WI			+0.150*(5)	
V.194 PF	+0.300 (1)	+0.235 (1)		
V.196 CM				-0.017*(7)
V.197 PSYCO			-0.161 (2)	-0.081*(4)
V.198 ACCONT	+0.147 (4)	+0.138 (2)	+0.382 (1)	+0.207 (1)
Constant	+0.591	1.073	1.620	1.651
Adjusted R^2	0.085	0.044	0.153	0.116
Standard error	0.802	0.832	0.879	0.811
Original mean	1.55	1.51	1.27	.52
Adjusted mean				
Thai	1.55	1.61	1.52	1.36
Chinese	1.49	1.51	1.43	1.34
Thai Muslim	1.41	1.46	1.27	1.10
Southern Thai Muslim	.89	1.08	.86	.52

NOTES: In the parentheses is the order of inclusion of the variable(s) in the equation(s). The asterisked variables are significant at .05 and the non-asterisked ones are significant at .01 level of significance.

contraception more than those who approve of high fertility. Also, those who feel that they have to pay a high (psychic) cost in using contraception will tend to use ineffective methods of contraception.

The use of effective contraception by the Southern Thai Muslims is positively related to wife's education and access to contraception and negatively related to psychic cost and husband's professional occupation (similar to Thai Muslims in other parts of the country), child mortality, religiosity and wife's ethnic affiliation. The findings imply that those who are more religious and strongly affiliated with their ethnic group and have experienced high child mortality are less likely to use effective contraception than those who have opposite characteristics.

In brief, the use of effective contraception of the four ethnic groups is affected by the one common factor of access to contraception and other factors unique to each ethnic group. There are other social and economic factors that uniquely affect the use of effective contraception of a particular ethnic group. The Thais are affected by income, perceived woman's role and household type; the Thai Muslims by ethnic fertility approval and wife's influence; and the Southern Thai Muslims by wife's ethnic fertility approval, wife's education and religiosity. However, there are also other factors affecting the use of effective contraception which are common to the two or three ethnic groups. For instance both the Thais and the Chinese are affected by perceived fecundity; the Chinese, the Thai Muslims and the Thais by gender balance; the Chinese and the Thai Muslims in the South and in other parts of the country by husband's professional occupation, and the Thai Muslims and the Southern Thai Muslims by psychic cost of contraception.

VI

CONCLUSION AND POLICY RECOMMENDATIONS

Analysis of factors affecting fertility and contraceptive use discussed in the previous chapter conclusively shows that ethnicity is unquestionably a significant variable in the study of fertility and family planning in Thailand. Ethnic groups significantly differ from one another not only in the level of fertility and use of effective contraception but also in the variables that significantly affect their fertility and contraceptive behaviour. Population policies and programmes must therefore be carefully formulated and designed for each ethnic group. This can only be achieved by a thorough study of the factors affecting fertility and family planning behaviour of each ethnic group. The findings of the research project suggest a number of policy implications.

The fact that all other ethnic groups have higher fertility than the Thais implies that, if the present ethnic composition of the country's population is to be maintained, more effort should be directed at reducing the high fertility of the Southern Thai Muslims, the Thai Muslims and the Chinese respectively. However, the aim of fertility reduction of the Thais should also not be disregarded as the Thais constitute the great majority of the country's population, and the success of slowing down population growth nationwide (which has been considered by the government a hindrance to national, social and economic progress) largely depends on fertility reduction of the Thais. The findings suggest that this can be done by making available family planning services to all ethnic groups as their use of effective contraception is affected by access to these services.

The findings on factors affecting fertility of the four ethnic groups further suggest ways and means to influence fertility behaviour of each ethnic group. Since the Chinese fertility is negatively influenced by wife's education and age at first marriage, a policy directed at improving the education of the Chinese women would not only have a negative impact on fertility but would also raise their age at first marriage which has, in turn, a negative effect on fertility.

Another factor that has policy implications for fertility reduction of the Chinese as well as of the other ethnic groups is gender balance. Data show that parents of all ethnic groups with a balanced sex composition of children have lower fertility than those with an unbalanced one. An attempt should be made to minimize the value that people place on sons, by educating all ethnic groups that boys and girls are equal and that both can equally contribute to the welfare of their families and society.

Among the Thai Muslims, data show that ethnic fertility approval is positively related to fertility. This implies that they consider high fertility not only appropriate for the group but also for themselves. Such an attitude constitutes a stumbling-block to any effort in reducing fertility of the group. Since this is an intricate issue, a programme directed at reducing fertility of the group should avoid activating the ethnic sentiments and should aim at increasing the well-being of the group.

It has also been found that fertility of the Southern Thai Muslims is positively affected by child mortality, similar to what has been found in other parts of the world. This implies that health programmes aiming at improving the health and welfare of mother and children will have a negative impact on fertility, and more of such programmes should be provided for the Southern Thai Muslims.

Insofar as family planning is concerned, analysis of data shows that the use of effective contraception by all ethnic groups is affected by their access to family planning services. The Thais and the Chinese use nearby services while the Muslims prefer distant to nearby services. Thus an attempt should be made to provide services to all ethnic groups so that all have better access to contraception.

The use of effective contraception by the Thais and the Chinese is also affected by other social and economic factors such as couple's income, perceived woman's role, gender balance and husband's occupation. The findings imply that the Thai and the Chinese men and women should be better educated in the roles of women and girls in the family and society.

It has also been found that ethnic fertility approval, ethnic affiliation, religiosity and psychic cost of contraception are negatively related to the use of effective contraception of the Thai Muslims and the Southern Thai Muslims. An attempt should be made to educate religious leaders in the problems of large families and to seek their co-operation in family planning campaigns. The process may take time and patience is required as it did with the Thai Buddhist monks. This will help reduce the psychic cost of using contraception among the Muslim minorities who want to practise family planning. All activities must be done with care and be constantly evaluated.

Appendix A

Matrices of Simple Correlation Coefficients

TABLE A.1

Matrix of Simple Correlation Coefficients of the Variables Used in Stepwise Regression Analysis of Fertility and Use of Effective Contraception of the Thais

Variable	V.82	V.176	V.115	V.178	V.179	V.53	V.75
V.176	0.09296						
V.115	0.19120	0.06935					
V.178	0.03123	-0.01804	-0.03889				
V.179	0.07401	0.06069	-0.06076	-0.01546			
V.53	-0.15660	0.06905	0.05758	-0.03128	-0.02147		
V.75	0.02628	-0.00441	-0.06476	0.06591	0.04326	-0.14085	
V.183	-0.01802	-0.09958	0.08956	-0.02753	-0.00432	0.11458	-0.12040
V.55	-0.22014	0.02592	0.02345	0.00961	-0.02555	0.36411	-0.17990
V.79	-0.02584	-0.10623	0.08032	0.03440	0.01637	0.05414	0.05276
V.184	-0.02211	-0.07501	0.04821	-0.02582	-0.05808	0.06405	-0.01607
V.185	0.07582	-0.09109	-0.05854	-0.01656	0.04972	-0.07446	0.06268
V.186	0.27392	0.16375	0.16860	-0.03449	0.04156	-0.01189	0.00313
V.187	-0.02380	0.06996	-0.05419	0.03906	0.00163	0.00463	-0.02976
V.49	0.11749	-0.10163	0.06879	-0.01458	0.03493	-0.06983	-0.01594
V.192	0.03086	0.01680	-0.01040	-0.04197	0.04004	-0.00475	-0.00393
V.193	-0.03283	0.01189	0.01781	-0.07113	-0.05960	0.03226	-0.02987
V.197	-0.02100	0.01116	-0.03947	-0.05585	0.03748	-0.06061	0.06820
V.198	0.00467	0.08144	0.12324	-0.01395	0.00222	0.00539	-0.02600
V.102	0.66706	-0.00837	0.06742	-0.00700	0.06516	-0.13230	0.02727
V.194	0.19711	0.15002	0.19593	0.00679	-0.02208	-0.05169	0.04633
V.195	0.21115	0.24715	0.04326	0.08087	0.04265	-0.13218	0.09254
V.196	0.06379	-0.40398	0.05374	-0.04297	-0.01198	-0.00451	-0.01338
V.51	0.06591	-0.10279	0.05853	-0.06746	0.00042	0.14598	-0.20030
V.152	-0.14694	-0.18645	-0.01715	-0.04042	0.00479	0.14261	-0.07329
V.180	0.68653	-0.27094	0.05135	0.07878	0.05000	-0.20178	0.07897

TABLE A.1 (cont'd)

V.183	V.55	V.79	V.184	V.185
.21303				
.51653	0.12604			
.00573	0.08662	0.00535		
.06222	-0.01527	0.09911	-0.06059	
.00142	-0.02918	-0.06353	-0.07778	0.04722
.00013	0.06506	0.00464	-0.08684	0.06548
.01049	-0.09106	0.02910	0.02041	-0.00429
.01256	0.08788	-0.02623	-0.07777	-0.04863
.05332	0.04586	0.02084	0.06557	-0.01172
.03756	-0.15518	-0.03713	-0.08833	0.08416
.02128	0.01946	0.00393	-0.05052	0.02114
.00884	-0.17086	-0.06972	0.03282	0.05753
.08990	-0.08261	0.03897	-0.05201	-0.05315
.07268	-0.21578	-0.05308	-0.15668	0.04650
.03307	-0.00728	0.03899	0.14603	0.01240
.08167	0.14856	-0.03903	0.05387	-0.02966
.16130	0.16766	0.08086	0.05368	0.06770
.08599	-0.23784	0.02512	-0.00620	0.18313

TABLE A.1 (cont'd)

Matrix of Simple Correlation Coefficients of the Variables Used in Stepwise Regression Analysis of Fertility and Use of Effective Contraception of the Thais

Variable	V.186	V.187	V.49	V.192	V.193	V.197
V.187	0.11008					
V.49	0.01429	-0.05203				
V.192	-0.00741	0.00302	-0.03048			
V.193	0.02335	-0.00692	-0.10488	-0.05456		
V.197	-0.04817	-0.00994	0.6621	-0.04423	-0.02424	
V.198	0.06910	-0.01790	-0.05567	-0.05668	0.04784	-0.0624
V.102	0.19022	-0.02791	0.06407	0.02524	-0.03961	0.0139
V.194	0.11419	0.00334	-0.00226	0.01602	-0.04605	-0.0415
V.195	0.20824	0.08717	-0.10013	-0.03898	0.03701	0.0936
V.196	0.03700	-0.10775	0.32823	0.00160	-0.07259	-0.0463
V.51	0.01885	-0.02391	-0.06597	-0.04208	0.07636	-0.0787
V.152	-0.09740	0.00903	0.10891	-0.01060	0.03243	-0.0711
V.180	0.16993	-0.04078	0.15158	-0.00424	-0.01078	-0.0250

TABLE A.1 (cont'd)

V.198	V.102	V.194	V.195	V.196	V.51
.00705					
.05771	0.12682				
.02199	0.11629	0.04110			
.07356	0.08735	0.03656	-0.49223		
.06844	0.06673	-0.03443	-0.09630	0.02982	
.02186	-0.10161	-0.03447	-0.28939	0.36360	0.10414
.00152	0.47873	0.03070	0.19243	0.07994	0.12383

TABLE A.2

Matrix of Simple Correlation Coefficients of the Variables Used in Stepwise Regression Analysis of Fertility and Use of Effective Contraception of the Chine

Variable	V.82	V.176	V.115	V.178	V.179	V.53
V.176	0.04483					
V.115	0.19975	0.06741				
V.178	0.00403	0.02970	-0.03564			
V.179	0.02157	-0.00748	-0.01870	0.08344		
V.53	-0.14508	0.06648	-0.03158	0.0	0.03516	
V.75	0.09926	0.03061	-0.07132	0.05652	0.0397	-0.017
V.183	0.10390	0.05188	0.03913	-0.08029	-0.03920	-0.026
V.55	-0.27425	0.06361	0.06404	-0.10969	0.02326	0.212
V.79	0.04887	-0.02263	0.02502	-0.09215	-0.00963	0.063
V.184	-0.04415	-0.00672	-0.03872	-0.02152	-0.00572	0.095
V.185	-0.01598	-0.09213	0.05430	0.00310	-0.07112	-0.009
V.186	0.31552	0.14531	0.10771	-0.00740	-0.03213	0.037
V.187	-0.07321	0.05028	0.00246	-0.01339	0.02822	0.088
V.49	0.12483	-0.26379	0.05183	0.01173	0.00476	-0.005
V.192	-0.03191	-0.02724	-0.01246	0.00760	-0.02407	0.015
V.193	-0.01792	0.07455	0.07333	-0.06557	0.03420	0.046
V.197	0.03979	0.00002	-0.05820	-0.05448	0.01588	0.045
V.198	0.04910	0.08952	0.12436	-0.00569	-0.04870	0.006
V.102	0.58592	0.01173	0.02794	0.02251	0.01650	-0.116
V.194	0.226-7	0.07584	0.14734	0.05459	-0.06147	0.014
V.195	0.19739	0.27005	0.02573	-0.02042	0.04259	-0.019
V.196	-0.00113	-0.46672	-0.03560	0.01570	-0.00085	-0.044
V.51	0.04589	-0.07820	0.02134	-0.12034	0.02082	0.128
V.152	-0.28025	-0.15057	-0.08207	-0.05751	-0.02735	0.049
V.180	0.69709	-0.28593	0.05842	-0.00563	0.01160	-0.162

TABLE A.2 (cont'd)

V.75	V.183	V.55	V.79	V.184	V.185
-0.07787					
-0.06015	0.07165				
0.02384	-0.19629	0.01232			
-0.02385	-0.02286	0.01590	-0.02033		
-0.03295	-0.01597	0.04789	-0.00411	-0.01123	
0.05783	-0.01044	-0.01113	0.00578	-0.01972	0.04445
0.02721	-0.03938	0.00183	0.11066	0.07782	0.03704
-0.06338	0.01341	-0.06499	0.01392	0.07834	-0.01277
0.00338	-0.04877	0.11585	0.00049	-0.05785	0.12287
-0.00163	0.02160	0.09460	0.02197	0.01928	-0.01896
-0.01714	-0.05051	-0.07447	-0.03306	-0.03677	-0.00534
0.01495	0.01352	0.04858	0.13110	-0.01431	0.05925
0.07632	0.06014	-0.18076	0.06338	-0.00603	-0.02506
0.02547	-0.01748	-0.03679	0.04735	0.03691	0.00820
0.15476	-0.04800	-0.08764	-0.01667	-0.10336	0.00835
-0.06437	-0.03215	0.00114	-0.00050	0.10770	0.03466
-0.14256	0.10874	0.05454	0.07729	0.00886	-0.01793
-0.05506	-0.00020	0.10212	-0.03640	0.06499	-0.02663
0.05975	0.10715	-0.30706	0.06061	-0.02609	0.04832

TABLE A.2 (cont'd)

Matrix of Simple Correlation Coefficients of the Variables Used in Stepwise Regression Analysis of Fertility and Use of Effective Contraception of the Chinese

Variable	V.186	V.187	V.49	V.192	V.193	V.197
V.187	0.11190					
V.49	0.04052	0.01223				
V.192	0.01409	0.01027	-0.01532			
V.193	0.03752	0.07685	-0.04858	-0.08605		
V.197	0.00131	-0.00194	0.01497	-0.02840	-0.08803	
V.198	0.06766	-0.00611	-0.04807	0.03456	0.05655	-0.14468
V.102	0.20091	-0.11299	0.12355	-0.01884	-0.08032	0.02783
V.194	0.09771	-0.02256	0.02078	0.02601	0.00072	-0.7248
V.195	0.16537	0.02301	-0.23044	0.01071	0.05583	0.00898
V.196	-0.02907	-0.08705	0.42246	0.03223	-0.16957	-0.04496
V.51	0.06068	0.00047	0.10565	-0.03345	0.04766	0.05548
V.152	-0.05771	0.02839	0.13742	-0.02235	-0.03761	-0.02451
V.180	0.12372	-0.07297	0.13274	-0.03822	0.01163	0.00652

TABLE A.2 (cont'd)

V.198	V.102	V.194	V.195	V.196	V.51
.03239					
.06026	0.13126				
.06433	0.08877	0.01568			
.12130	0.09170	0.03522	-0.50958		
.07654	0.01758	-0.05232	-0.05508	0.02937	
.06338	-0.11517	-0.09728	-0.33494	0.41353	0.12189
.00422	0.41350	0.04831	0.16130	-0.01359	0.05226

TABLE A.3

Matrix of Simple Correlation Coefficients of the Variables Used in Stepwise Regression Analysis of Fertility and Use of Effective Contraception of the Thai Muslims

Variable	V.82	V.176	V.115	V.178	V.179	V.53
V.176	0.11696					
V.115	0.01469	-0.02593				
V.178	0.08076	0.05638	-0.01732			
V.179	0.11442	0.11499	-0.07608	0.09226		
V.53	-0.15963	0.01717	0.04572	-0.08338	-0.06301	
V.75	0.12570	0.11035	-0.08476	0.10059	0.11252	-0.133
V.183	-0.01365	-0.09530	0.09658	-0.09864	-0.06287	0.098
V.55	-0.25717	-0.05908	0.06625	0.00562	-0.06559	0.381
V.79	-0.08033	-0.08082	0.03145	-0.00052	0.04479	0.158
V.184	0.05508	0.03769	-0.03736	-0.04854	0.04539	-0.042
V.185	0.09358	-0.08944	-0.05431	0.04953	0.07442	0.024
V.186	0.22257	0.30179	0.12314	0.06467	0.07696	-0.026
V.187	-0.02104	0.07688	0.01206	-0.07279	-0.01090	-0.009
V.49	0.13105	-0.06456	0.06311	-0.02163	0.02596	-0.047
V.192	0.02576	0.00854	-0.09343	0.06330	0.00977	0.067
V.193	0.03888	0.00893	0.07934	-0.03001	-0.02532	-0.023
V.197	-0.04437	0.07947	-0.19028	0.04646	0.09448	-0.069
V.198	0.02852	0.00360	0.31794	0.00254	0.06019	0.031
V.102	0.42032	0.08522	0.04668	0.08431	0.05765	-0.035
V.194	0.30208	0.15112	0.03161	0.01958	0.10501	-0.048
V.195	0.17378	0.34222	0.03545	0.04592	0.08115	-0.134
V.196	0.05309	-0.30430	-0.00400	-0.00889	0.03495	-0.001
V.51	0.03788	-0.15669	0.08518	-0.10950	-0.13240	0.129
V.152	-0.20545	-0.20644	0.03944	-0.08469	-0.04587	0.171
V.180	0.69894	-0.15636	-0.00474	0.02217	0.01041	-0.158

TABLE A.3 (cont'd)

V.75	V.183	V.55	V.79	V.184	V.185
-0.14667					
-0.14323	0.10695				
0.00854	0.35583	0.12933			
0.01122	-0.02473	-0.08656	-0.06253		
0.08972	-0.02841	-0.04151	-0.04588	-0.00391	
0.05201	0.02870	-0.04133	-0.03985	-0.00764	-0.00377
-0.00270	0.01389	-0.00533	0.00616	0.02348	-0.04015
-0.03323	0.02655	-0.07440	-0.05523	-0.06410	0.06027
0.04718	-0.05298	-0.11450	-0.03969	0.00872	0.04263
-0.02245	0.03279	-0.01415	0.04704	-0.00792	-0.06052
0.00889	-0.05217	-0.02192	0.07474	0.02193	0.06491
0.02747	0.06186	0.05769	0.06030	-0.00866	-0.03834
0.11288	0.06675	-0.08428	-0.04903	-0.00335	0.14898
0.08833	-0.08014	-0.06571	-0.02625	0.06728	0.02686
0.10856	-0.05995	-0.16981	-0.07223	0.01982	-0.03154
-0.01483	-0.08670	-0.01389	-0.01617	-0.03070	0.12227
-0.26997	0.17266	0.11476	0.07359	0.03294	0.00681
-0.07483	0.08822	0.16317	0.04335	-0.01331	0.02950
0.05148	0.05980	-0.25837	-0.05028	0.00466	0.10803

TABLE A.3 (cont'd)
Matrix of Simple Correlation Coefficients of the
Variables Used in Stepwise Regression Analysis of
Fertility and Use of Effective Contraception of the Thai Muslims

Variable	V.186	V.187	V.49	V.192	V.193	V.197
V.187	0.08948					
V.49	-0.06729	-0.04834				
V.192	-0.07503	-0.07154	0.05137			
V.193	-0.00535	0.09074	-0.04253	-0.11193		
V.197	-0.00215	0.05135	-0.12823	-0.03064	-0.03469	
V.198	0.11450	0.08313	-0.03126	-0.10142	-0.01975	-0.0390
V.102	0.10034	-0.05824	0.05020	0.03440	-0.05600	0.0122
V.194	0.14707	-0.03441	0.06663	0.05991	-0.05762	-0.0911
V.195	0.33836	0.07880	-0.07021	-0.06915	0.02592	0.0414
V.196	0.07717	-0.09644	0.19885	0.01966	-0.10655	0.0126
V.51	-0.04636	-0.03034	-0.03617	-0.03041	0.01658	-0.0658
V.152	-0.17884	-0.03784	0.11144	0.09591	-0.09952	-0.0463
V.180	0.15406	0.00297	0.14569	-0.01203	0.06225	-0.0643

TABLE A.3 (cont'd)

V.198	V.102	V.194	V.195	V.196	V.51
0.02279					
0.01609	0.18201				
0.04560	0.09844	0.13136			
0.03145	0.04340	-0.03081	-0.32959		
0.00063	-0.01346	0.00780	-0.09862	-0.05790	
0.00169	-0.08521	-0.03776	-0.32458	0.22987	0.17598
0.03677	0.33038	0.11392	0.15940	0.03727	0.15532

TABLE A.4

Matrix of Simple Correlation Coefficients of the Variables Used in Stepwise Regression Analysis of Fertility and Use of Effective Contraception of the Southern Thai Muslims

Variable	V.82	V.176	V.115	V.178	V.179	V.53
V.176	0.13630					
V.115	0.00660	0.10043				
V.178	0.11776	-0.00057	-0.14511			
V.179	0.04500	0.00037	-0.01144	0.03651		
V.53	-0.29794	-0.07352	0.16882	-0.24598	0.03677	
V.75	0.07158	-0.04500	-0.16451	0.09759	0.00401	-0.26820
V.183	0.04909	-0.08172	-0.04463	0.05840	-0.00949	0.10854
V.55	-0.39386	-0.02027	0.19509	-0.21992	0.01843	0.57759
V.79	0.09094	-0.00600	0.01842	0.11986	-0.01116	0.07916
V.184	0.11697	-0.02778	-0.05132	0.03358	0.07469	-0.10650
V.185	0.01257	-0.03206	-0.06141	-0.09054	-0.02708	0.01751
V.186	0.25884	0.15576	0.04779	0.00717	-0.03285	-0.07747
V.187	-0.04336	0.04081	0.04926	0.01572	0.02145	0.04699
V.49	0.07948	-0.20044	-0.04736	0.01286	-0.05290	-0.04875
V.192	-0.01238	-0.06083	-0.03200	-0.03922	-0.01594	0.14304
V.193	0.00086	-0.04212	-0.05032	-0.02128	0.02227	-0.01704
V.197	0.01205	-0.00629	-0.14451	0.02156	-0.05759	0.03322
V.198	-0.05892	0.02001	0.23639	-0.01252	0.01190	0.08982
V.102	0.35481	0.09665	-0.03802	-0.00734	0.02724	-0.15138
V.194	0.34996	0.17262	-0.00897	0.11864	0.07479	-0.14080
V.195	0.17882	0.27413	-0.05546	0.12989	-0.02341	-0.20901
V.196	0.04284	-0.54447	-0.06881	0.02089	0.04057	0.04173
V.51	0.24966	0.02134	-0.01232	0.04275	-0.03313	0.02646
V.152	-0.09136	-0.32362	0.01739	-0.09819	-0.01380	0.22718
V.180	0.69834	-0.12810	-0.08807	0.16262	0.02960	-0.35185

TABLE A.4 (cont'd)

V.75	V.183	V.55	V.79	V.184	V.185
.05888					
.21205	0.14627				
.01716	0.52484	0.07588			
01145	0.00869	-0.07426	-0.04380		
00393	-0.00376	0.05636	0.03441	-0.12662	
00806	-0.02729	-0.12739	0.05411	0.03539	0.03713
02374	-0.01036	0.04887	0.01972	0.12285	-0.01931
02511	-0.05344	-0.05319	-0.02949	-0.03631	-0.03443
06390	0.15366	0.12918	0.07736	0.01028	-0.01918
00500	-0.03443	-0.05912	0.03105	0.05304	0.05570
07402	0.04217	-0.03477	0.02844	0.01871	0.04700
17017	0.03507	0.14250	0.15896	-0.07274	0.07313
11689	-0.02158	-0.19605	0.07565	0.00973	0.01119
02846	0.01071	-0.11196	0.02421	0.14049	-0.15019
12032	-0.01573	-0.15432	-0.00040	0.07393	-0.01133
02578	0.04587	-0.00810	0.02044	0.06156	-0.00637
14405	-0.05815	-0.09392	-0.04504	0.01534	0.00325
06752	0.13241	0.19906	0.08465	0.01207	0.02747
20241	0.08759	-0.4752	0.08901	0.05990	0.04768

TABLE A.4 (cont'd)

Matrix of Simple Correlation Coefficients of the Variables Used in Stepwise Regression Analysis of Fertility and Use of Effective Contraception of the Southern Thai Muslims

Variable	V.186	V.187	V.49	V.192	V.193	V.197
V.187	-0.01570					
V.49	0.08440	-0.12095				
V.192	0.03693	-0.08036	0.02596			
V.193	-0.04097	0.08299	-0.02020	-0.04298		
V.197	-0.01079	-0.00924	-0.01505	0.02719	-0.12083	
V.198	-0.04450	0.08418	-0.01620	-0.00826	0.03426	-0.170
V.102	0.10642	-0.07920	0.02404	-0.04582	0.00630	-0.001
V.194	0.11769	-0.02028	0.06583	0.05857	0.00847	0.048
V.195	0.14128	0.03195	-0.13037	-0.03451	-0.07168	0.048
V.196	-0.02514	-0.14362	0.42387	0.10121	0.09884	-0.028
V.51	0.04945	-0.04290	0.05268	-0.15730	0.06664	-0.035
V.152	-0.05314	-0.08912	0.22155	0.12930	0.01363	0.013
V.180	0.19304	-0.07612	0.09990	-0.00164	0.03347	0.018

TABLE A.4 (cont'd)

V.198	V.102	V.194	V.195	V.196	V.51
.04737					
.08270	0.07915				
.05881	0.08320	0.12893			
.06302	0.00711	-0.02427	-0.42921		
.01003	0.07408	0.05033	-0.08815	0.05916	
.08965	-0.08256	-0.06388	-0.31670	0.55992	0.15431
.13293	0.26959	0.12391	0.20237	0.03555	0.10772

APPENDIX 1A

Notations on Variables

WEAFF = Wife's ethnic affiliation

AGE = Wife's current age

WED = Wife's education

FEM = Female employment

AFM = Wife's age at first marriage

HOCC = Husband's occupation

PWR = Perceived woman's role

HDOM = Husband's dominance

CINC = Couple's income

RELI = Religiosity

MBF = Months of breastfeeding

SONPREF = Son preference

CM = Child mortality

EFERA = Ethnic fertility approval

PSYCO = Psychic cost of contraception

DFS = Desired family size

CEB = Cumulative fertility or total number of children ever born

CONTRA = Contraceptive practice

RFER = Recent fertility or fertility during the past 5 years

HPROF = Husband's occupation -- professional

HFARM = Husband's occupation -- farming

HUNCL = Husband's occupation -- unclassified

APPENDIX 1B

Specification of Variables Used in the Multi-variate Analysis

CEB = Total number of children ever born

UEM = Use of effective contraceptive method

Effective method = 2
Traditional method = 1

Effective methods = Pill, IUD, Sterilization, Condom, Injectables.

Traditional methods = Douche, Rhythm, Withdrawal, Abstention, Other (Herb, etc.)

RF = Recent Fertility, i.e., number of children ever born within the last five years

EG = Ethnic group

Chinese = 1
Thai = 2
Thai Muslim = 3
Southern Thai Muslim = 4

EAFF = Ethnic fertility affiliation

Summation of the following:

(1) School

Ever attended own ethnic/religious school = 2
No schooling = 1
Never attended own ethnic/religious school = 0

(2) Associations

Ever belong to own ethnic associations = 2
No association = 1
Belong to other ethnic association = 0

(3) Friends

All friends from own ethnic group = 2
No friends at all = 1
Friends from at least some other ethnic group = 0

EFERA = Ethnic fertility approval

Summation of the following:

(1) Better socio-economic position with many or few children

Many	= 3
Does not matter	= 2
Few	= 1

(2) Whether your ethnic group's families have too many, too few or just the right number of children

Too many	= 1
Right number	= 2
Too few	= 3

(3) An ethnic group can only be strong if there are many of them

True	= 3
Partly true	= 2
False	= 1

HED = Husband's education

Level of education attained in years.

WED = Wife's education

Level of education attained in years.

HOC = Husband's occupation

Professional	= 1
Services/Production	= 2
Farm	= 3
Unclassified	= 4

CINC = Couple's income in 10 categorical scale

PWR = Perceived woman's role

Summation of the following:

(1) A girl becomes fully a woman only when she bears her own children

Strongly agree	= 5
Slightly agree	= 4
Neutral	= 3

Slightly disagree = 2
Strongly disagree = 1

(2) A woman should devote a lot of time satisfying her husband (Score as above)

(3) Is it a good idea or a bad idea for a woman to work outside the home after marriage? Do you approve of a woman working even if her husband's earnings are adequate?

5 = bad idea to work outside
4 = indifferent to the first question but no to the second question
3 = indifferent to the first question but yes to the second
2 = good idea on the first but no to the second
1 = good idea on the first but yes to the second

HOC = Husband's occupation

Professional	= 1
Services/Production	= 2
Farm	= 3
Unclassified	= 4

CINC = Couple's income in 10 categorical scale

PWR = Perceived woman's role

Summation of the following

(1) A girl becomes fully a woman only when she bears her own children

Strongly agree	= 5
Slightly agree	= 4
Neutral	= 3
Slightly disagree	= 2
Strongly disagree	= 1

(2) A woman should devote a lot of time satisfying her husband (Score as above)

(3) Is it a good idea or a bad idea for a woman to work outside the home after marriage? Do you approve of a woman working even if her husband's earnings are adequate?

5 = bad idea to work outside
4 = indifferent to the first question but no to the second question
3 = indifferent to the first question but yes to the second
2 = good idea on the first but no to the second
1 = good idea on the first but yes to the second

SPIN = Spouse interation

Whether you can confide in or share worries with your spouse all the time, most of the time, sometimes, or seldom.

All the time = 4
Most of the time = 3
Sometimes = 2
Seldom = 1

HELI = Religiosity

Summation of the following:

(1) How often do you pray?

Several times a day = 6
Once a day = 5
At least once a week = 4
At least once a month = 3
Less than once a month = 2
Never = 1

(2) How often do you attend religious services or ceremonies

(Score as above)

(3) How important is religion in your daily life

Very important = 3
Quite important = 2
Not important = 1

MBF = Months of breastfeeding of the most recent child

FEM = Female employment

Never worked = 0
Work at home = 1
Work nearby = 2
Work far away = 3

GENB = Gender balance

No children = 0
Balance = 1
More sons = 2
More daughters = 3

SONPRE = Son preference

If you were to have exactly three children altogether, how many would you want to be boys and how many to be girls?

3 girls = 1
2 girls, 1 boy = 2
Either sex = 3
2 boys, 1 girl = 4
3 boys = 5

HTYPE = Household type

Nuclear (including unrelated persons, e.g., servants/boarders, etc) = 1
Joint with one couple = 2
Joint with more than one couple = 3

HDOM = Husband dominance

If you were to disagree about how many children to have, whose opinion would be more important; yours or your (husband's/wife's)

Husband = 2
Wife = 1

DFS = Desired family size

= Number of living children plus number of additional children desired

FECUN = Perceived fecundity

Relative to other couples of the same age, how difficult is it for (you/your wife) to become pregnant?

Impossible/Infecund = 0
Very difficult = 1
A little difficult = 2
Fairly easy = 3
Very easy = 4

ACCONT = Access to contraception

How long would it take you to go from your house to the nearest place or person to get supplies or other family planning help, if you needed it, (in minutes)

PSYCOS = Psychic cost of contraception obtained by adding all six scores from six questions on the disliked characteristics of contraception

Very important = 3
Fairly important = 2
Not important = 1

The questions are:

(1) A contraceptive method that may affect your/your wife's health

(2) A method that is unpleasant to use

(3) If it is irreversible

(4) If it requires examination (of your wife) by a man

(5) If it requires surgery

(6) If it is against your religion

CMOR = Child mortality, i.e., number of children died after birth

BIBLIOGRAPHY

Aziz, Datin Nor Laily and others. Culture and Fertility Study Country Report -- Malaysia. Malaysia: National Family Planning Board, 1978.

Bean, Frank D. and Charles H. Wood. "Ethnic Variations in the Relationship between Income and Fertility". Demography 11 (1974): 629-40.

Bean, Frank D. and J.P. Marcum. "Differential fertility and the minority-group status hypothesis -- assessment and review". In Demography of Racial and Ethnic Groups, ed. Frank D. Bean and W.P. Frisbie. New York: Academic Press, 1977.

Berelson, Bernard. "Ethnicity and fertility: what and so what". In Zero Population Growth -- For Whom? Differential Fertility and Minority Group Survival, ed. Milton Himmelfarb and Victor Baras, pp. 74-118. Westport, Connecticut: Greenword Press, Inc., 1978.

Bongaarts, John. "A framework for analyzing the proximate determinants of fertility". Population and Development Review 4, no. 1 (1978): 105-32.

Boulier, Bryan and Mark R. Rosenzweig. "Age, biological factors, and socioeconomic determinants of fertility: a new measure of cumulative fertility for use in the socioeconomic analysis of family size". Demography 15 (1978): 487-97.

Bulatao, Rodolfo A. Ethnic Attitudes and Five Philippine Cities. Quezon City: Social Research Laboratory, University of the Philippines, 1973.

Bunnag, Saranya. Social and Economic Factors Affecting Desire for 2-Child Family Among Different Ethnic Groups in Southern

Thailand. Faculties of Management Science, Prince of Songkla University, 1982.

Chang, Chen-Tung. Fertility Transition in Singapore. Singapore: Singapore University Press, 1974.

Cho, Lee-Jay and Robert D. Retherford. "Comparative analysis of recent fertility trends in East Asia". In Proceedings of the International Population Conference. Liege: International Union for the Scientific Study of Population, 1973.

Clignet, Remi and Joyce A. Sween. "Ethnicity and fertility: implications for population programs in Africa". Africa 48, no. 1 (1978): 47-65.

Coale, Ansley J. "The demographic transition". In International Population Conference, Vol. 1. Liege: International Union for the Scientific Study of Population, 1973.

______. "The demographic transition". Paper presented at the Conference on Fertility Transition, Kyoto, December, 1975.

Davis, Kingsley and Judith Blake. "Social structure and fertility: an analytic framework". Economic Development and Cultural Change 4, no. 4 (1956): 211-35.

Day, Lincoln. "Nativity and ethnocentrism: some relationships suggested by an analysis of Catholic-Protestant differentials". Population Studies 22 (1968): 27-50.

Goldscheider, Calvin and Peter R. Uhlenberg. "Minority group status and fertility". American Journal of Sociology 74 no. 4 (1969): 361-73.

Goldstein, Sidney. "Religious fertility differentials in Thailand, 1960". Population Studies 14, no. 3 (1970): 325-37.

Gurak, Douglas T. "Sources of ethnic fertility differences: an examination of five minority groups". Social Science Quarterly 59, no. 2 (1978): 295-310.

Himmelfarb, Milton and Victor Baras, eds. Zero Population Growth -- For Whom? Differential Fertility and Minority Group Survival. Westport, Connecticut: Greenwood Press, Inc., 1978.

Jiobu, R. and H. Marshall. "Minority status and family size: a comparison of explanations". Population Studies 31, no. 3 (1977): 509-17.

Johnson, Nan E. "Minority-group status and the fertility of black Americans, 1970: a new look". Paper prepared for the annual meeting of the Population Association of America, Philadelphia, Pennsylvania, April 26-28, 1979.

Jones, Gavin and Yanee Soonthornthum. "Fertility and contraception in the rural south of Thailand". Bangkok: Manpower Planning Division, National Economic Development Board, 1971.

Kennedy, Robert E., Jr. "Minority group status and fertility: the Irish". American Sociological Review 38 (February 1973): 85-96.

Lopez, David E. and Georges Sabagh. "Untangling structural and normative aspects of the minority status-fertility hypothesis". American Journal of Sociology 83 (May 1978): 1491-497.

Lorimer, Frank. "General Theory". In Culture and Human Fertility, ed. Frank Lorimer and others, pp. 14-251. Paris: UNESCO, 1954.

Marshall, Harvey and James Sinnott. "Urban structure and black/white fertility differential". Social Science Quarterly 52 (1971): 558-601.

Marshall, Harvey H. and Robert M. Jiobu. "An alternate test of the minority status and fertility relation". Pacific Sociological Review 21, no. 2 (1978): 221-37.

Marshall, John F. and Steven Polgar, eds. Culture, Natality, and Family Planning. Chapel Hill: Carolina Population Center, 1976.

Nag, Moni. Factors Affecting Human Fertility in Nonindustrial Societies: A Cross-Cultural Study. Yale University Publications in Anthropology 66. New Haven: Yale University, 1962.

Nag, Moni, ed. Population and Social Organization. The Hague: Monton Publishers, 1975.

Pohlmann, Vernon C. and Robert H. Walsh. "Black minority racial status and fertility in the United States, 1970". Sociological Focus 8 (1975): 97-109.

Polgar, Steven, ed. Culture and Population. Cambridge, Mass.: Schenkman, 1971.

Prachuabmoh, Visid, John Knodel, and J. Oscar Alers. "Preference for sons, desire for additional children, and family planning in Thailand". Institute of Population Studies, Paper No. 16. Bangkok: Chulalongkorn University, 1974.

Prasithrathsint, Suchart. "Family Planning of the Rural Women in Thailand". Journal of Social Sciences 9, no. 1 (1972): 63-71.

______. "Family Planning of the Rural Women in Thailand". Ramathibodhi, 2, no. 5 (1971): 28-38.

______. "Implications of Sex Preferences for Prospective Children on the Fertility and of the Thai Rural Families." Ramathihodhi 3, no. 4 (1972): 138-55.

______. "Regional Socio-Economic Inequalities and Population Migration". Journal of Population Education (1973).

______. Fertility Threshold Values of Income and Education in Thailand. Bangkok: National Institute of Development Administration, 1979.

Prasithrathsint, Suchart, Likhit Dhiravegin, and Chavalit Siripirom. Culture and Fertility in Thailand: A Cross-National Comparative Study. Thailand: Mahidol University, 1978.

Prompaichit, Suttipong. "The Impact of the Religions Beliefs and Customs of the Thai Muslims in Southern Thailand on Fertility". In Fertility and Development Interactions in Thailand, ed. Suchart Prasithrathsint. Rayong: Sahapomkanpim, 1982.

Ritchey, Neal P. "The effect of minority group status on fertility: a re-examination of concepts". Population Studies 29 (July 1975): 249-57.

Roberts, Robert E. and Eun Sul Lee. "Minority group status and fertility revisited". American Journal of Sociology 80, no. 2 (1974): 503-23.

Saw Swee-Hock. "Fertility differentials in early postwar Malaya". Demography 42 no. 2 (1967): 641-56.

______. Singapore Population in Transition. Philadelphia: University of Pennsylvania Press, 1970.

Sly, David F. "Minority-group status and fertility: an extension of Goldscheider and Uhlenberg". American Journal of Sociology 76 (1970): 443-59.

Smith, Peter C. "Regional and urban-rural data on cumulative fertility: May, 1973". Population Institute Research Note No. 29. Manila: University of the Philippines, 1974.

______. "Fertility and nuptiality: the local-area mosaic". In A Demographic Path to Modernity, ed. Wilhelm Flieger and Peter C. Smith, pp. 201-33. Quezon City: The University of the Philippines Press, 1975.

Snyder, D.W. "Tribal affiliation and fertility: a note". Population Studies 29, no. 1 (1975): 151-54.

Stinner, William F. "Modernization, marriage and childbearing: a synthesis of research findings". In A Demographic Path to Modernity, ed. Wilhelm Flieger and Perer C. Smith pp. 4-37. Quezon City: The University of the Philippines Press, 1975.

Stinner, William F. and Paul Douglas Mader. "Government policy and personal family planning approval in conflict settings: the case of the Muslim minority in the southern Philippines". Population Studies 29, no. 1 (1975): 53-59.

Stokes, C. Shannon, Kelly W. Carder, and Jack C. Smith. "Race, education, and fertility: a comparison of black-white reproductive behavior". Phylon 38 (June 1977).

Stycos, J. Mayone. Human Fertility in Latin America. Ithaca: Cornell University Press, 1968.

______. "Opinion, idealogy, and population problems -- some sources of domestic and foreign opposition to birth control". In Rapid Population Growth, ed. National Academy of Sciences, pp. 551-54. Baltimore: Johns Hopkins Press, 1971.

Suits, Daniel B., Andrew Mason, and Louis Chan. "Spline functions fitted by standard regression methods". The Review of Economics and Statistics 60, no. 1 (1978): 132-39.

Suparlan, Parsudi and Hananto Sigit. Culture and Fertility: Indonesia. Indonesia: LEKNAS, 1978.

Suvipakit, Soontaree. "A pilot study of family health in Thai Muslim communities in South Thailand". Yala Project, Report No. 1. Bangkok: The National Research Council, 1969.

United Nations. The Determinants and Consequences of Population Trends. Vol. 1 (1973), New York.

Van de Walle, Etienne. "The view from the past: population change and group survival". In Zero Population Growth -- For Whom?, Differential Fertility and Minority Group Survival, ed. Milton Himmelfarb and Victor Baras, pp. 6-25. Westport, Connecticut: Greenwood Press, Inc., 1978.